D0690308

Ellie Herman's

Pilates
Workbook
on the Ball

Ellie Herman's

Pilates
Workbook
on the Ball

Illustrated step-by-step guide

photography by Andy Mogg

Ulysses Press

Copyright © 2004 Ulysses Press. All rights reserved. No part of this publication may be repro-
duced, stored in a retrieval system, or transmitted in any form or by any means without the prior
written permission of the publisher, nor be otherwise circulated in any form of binding or cover
other than that in which it is published and without a similar condition being imposed on the sub-
sequent purchaser.

Published in the United States by
Ulysses Press
P.O. Box 3440
Berkeley, CA 94703
www.ulyssespress.com

Library of Congress Card Number 2003115848
ISBN 1-56975-388-1

Printed in Canada by Transcontinental Printing

10 9 8 7 6 5 4 3 2 1

Editorial/Production	Lynette Ubois, Steven Schwartz, Claire Chun, James Meetze, Lily Chou, Kate Allen
Interior Design	Sarah Levin
Cover Design	Leslie Henriques, Sarah Levin
Photography	Andy Mogg
Models	Ellie Herman, Alisa Michelle, Daniel Gregori

Distributed in the United States by Publishers Group West
and in Canada by Raincoast Books

Please Note
This book has been written and published strictly for informational purposes, and in no way
should be used as a substitute for consultation with health care professionals. You should not
consider educational material herein to be the practice of medicine or to replace consultation with
a physician or other medical practitioner. The author and publisher are providing you with information in this work so that you can have the knowledge and can choose, at your own risk, to act
on that knowledge. The author and publisher also urge all readers to be aware of their health sta-
tus and to consult health care professionals before beginning any health program.

I would like to dedicate this book to all my wonderful students,
who eventually become my teachers

contents

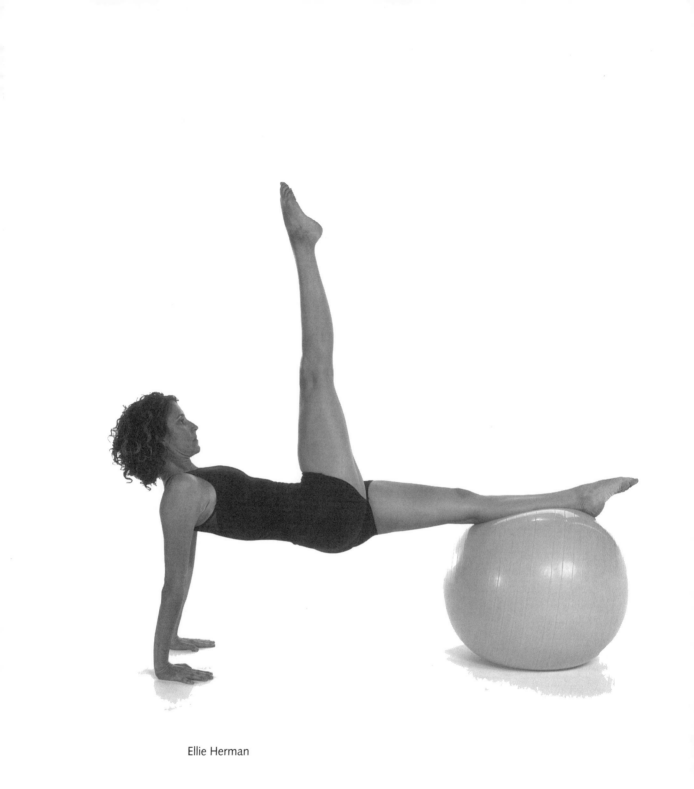

Ellie Herman

introduction

My torrid romance with Pilates began many years ago when I was a professional dancer and choreographer with my own dance company in San Francisco. To supplement my paltry income and to satisfy my desire for edgy experience, I decided to try my hand as a professional wrestler. My career as "Ruth Less" was cut short by a serious knee injury, which occurred during a tag-team match. At the time I cursed myself for being so stupid: How could I have taken my body for granted, especially being a dancer. I thought for sure my life as a dancer was over. But then I learned about St. Francis Hospital DanceMedicine in San Francisco, where I ventured to heal myself with this mysterious thing called Pilates. I was lucky enough to be put under the care of Elizabeth Larkham, one of the superstars of modern Pilates. After months of Pilates rehabilitation and no surgery (normally advisable after an anterior cruciate ligament tear), I returned to dancing only to realize that, to my surprise, I was a much better dancer than before my injury. Pilates had not only allowed me to return to jumping, leaping, and twirling, it had actually improved my technique, control, balance,

and core strength. At this moment, I became a Pilates convert.

I then moved to New York City, where I briefly attended the Masters program in dance at New York University. The best thing about my short stay at NYU was the morning Pilates mat class with Kathy Grant, one of the disciples of Joe Pilates. She taught me how depth and creativity could be brought to the Pilates method, while getting me out of the mounting hip pain that was due to the ballet classes I was taking every day. These Pilates classes inspired me to pursue Pilates teacher training with Romana Kyranowska, another of Joe Pilates original students.

I returned to San Francisco in 1992 and continued my study of Pilates with Jennifer Stacey and Carol Appel of Body Kinetics. The following year I opened my own studio in my live/work loft in the Mission district of San Francisco. The studio expanded so much over the years that we moved to a bigger building, with two full floors dedicated to Pilates-based fitness, rehabilitation, teacher training, continuing education, and complementary medicine. As the demand for good Pilates

instruction grew, so did my business, and I opened a second studio in Oakland, California, in 2001. Somewhere during all this expansion I managed to earn a Master of Science degree in Acupuncture & Chinese Herbal Medicine.

I've now taught Pilates for over ten years and have developed a unique language with which to communicate the essence of the Pilates method. Please see the section entitled Ellie Herman's Pilates Alphabet for my particular Pilates terms and concepts, used throughout the book. I hope these tools help you to understand the subtleties of Pilates in both a physical and conceptual way.

I continually strive to integrate my studies and expand my approach to bringing balance back to the body. As part of my ongoing interest in Pilates innovation, I have developed a new piece of Pilates equipment called the Pilates Springboard, an inexpensive and space-saving variation of the Wall Unit/ Cadillac. You can find out more about the Pilates Springboard on my website www.ellie.net, where you can also find information on my other upcoming projects, including a video you can use with this book.

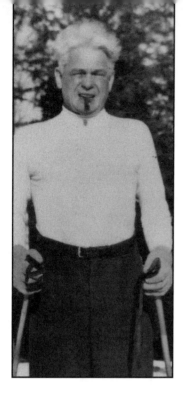

the story of Joe

The story goes that Joseph Hubertus Pilates was born in Germany in 1880, and as a child suffered from asthma and a sunken chest. He spent his life obsessed with restoring his health and body condition. Over his lifetime, he overcame his frailties and became an accomplished athlete. He loved skiing, diving, gymnastics, yoga, and boxing. There are famous pictures of the man looking extremely fit well into his 70s—doing Pilates exercises in the snow.

Originally Joe developed a series of mat exercises designed to build abdominal strength and body control. He then built various pieces of equipment to enhance the results of his expanding repertoire of exercises. His idea behind building the equipment was to replace himself as a spotter for his clients.

How He Invented the Pilates Equipment

Stationed in an English internment camp during WWI, Pilates rigged springs above hospital beds, allowing patients to rehabilitate while lying on their backs. This particular set-up later evolved into the Cadillac, one of the main pieces of Pilates equipment. He then developed over 20 contraptions—some of which look a little like medieval torture devices—constructed of wood and metal piping, using a variable combination of pulleys, straps, bars, boxes, and springs.

In his words, the Pilates method "develops the body uniformly, corrects wrong postures, restores physical vitality, invigorates the mind, and elevates the spirit." Joe was way ahead of his time, viewing the body holistically and emphasizing the body working as a whole unit.

Through the decades, Pilates developed over 500 exercises, which he originally called Contrology, but have since come to be known as the Pilates method.

In 1923 Joseph Pilates emigrated to the United States, settling in New York City, where he opened a studio on Eighth Avenue in Manhattan and started training and rehabilitating professional dancers (George Balanchine and Martha Graham were two of his students).

Joe's Legacy

The original Eighth Avenue Pilates studio in Manhattan is where the first generation of teachers were trained, including Romana Kyranowska, Kathy Grant, Ron Fletcher, Eve Gentry, Carola Trier, Mary Bowen, and

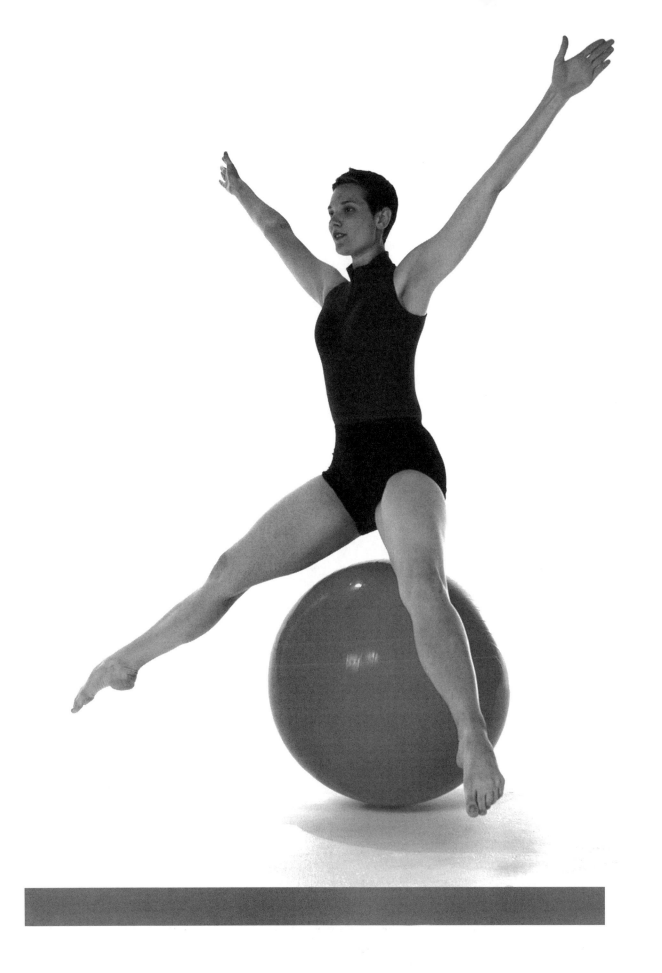

Bruce King. These protégés branched out and opened studios around the country, changing the method based on their own individual backgrounds and philosophies. For the following 50 years or so, the Pilates method has been passed down through many more generations of teachers and has transformed a great deal along the way. Some of the New York teachers claim to hold truest to the "original" method, but many creative individuals have brought their own insights to improve upon some of the more antiquated views of the body. Joe was a trailblazer, but his ideas can be improved upon. Even within his lifetime, he evolved his repertoire and changed his approach to better attain his desired results.

Pilates Now

Today, the Pilates method consists of a repertoire of over 500 exercises to be done on a mat or on one of the many pieces of equipment Joseph Pilates invented. The exercises are usually done in a series organized by levels: beginning, intermediate, advanced, and super-advanced. Pilates exercises as a whole develop strong abdominal, back, butt, and deep postural muscles to support the skeletal system and act as what Pilates called the "powerhouse" of the body. The Pilates method works to strengthen the center, lengthen the spine, increase body awareness, build muscle tone, and gain flexibility. The Pilates method is also an excellent rehabilitation system for back, knee, hip, shoulder, and repetitive stress injuries. Pilates addresses the body as a whole, correcting the body's asymmetries and chronic weaknesses to prevent re-injury and bring the body back into balance. As Joe used to say, "after 10 sessions you'll notice a difference, after 20 sessions other people will notice a difference, after 30 sessions you'll have a whole new body."

Pilates and the Ball

The ball is not a piece of Pilates equipment, nor was it used, as far as I know, by Joseph Pilates in his original studio. The Physioball®, the official term for the large ball, was originally developed by physical therapists in Switzerland to allow spine injury patients to do aerobic conditioning (bouncing). Physical therapists the world over continue to use the ball for all kinds of rehabilitation.

Like most physical therapists, we Pilates instructors also love the ball. Why? Because in addition to being a colorful, fun accessory to bounce on, it also acts as an excellent tool to reinforce many of the essential elements of the Pilates method: core stabilization, balance, and control.

For this book, I have gone through all the Pilates mat and reformer exercises and reinvented them using the ball. The ball provides different functions depending on what exercise you're doing. In certain exercises the ball acts as an incredibly unstable surface upon which you must stabilize yourself (e.g., the Plank, the One-Legged Bridge). In other exercises, the ball acts as an extra weight, either in your arms or between your legs, that adds an extra conditioning element to the exercise (e.g., the Dead Hang Fold). Other times, the ball provides a surface to sit and roll around on to facilitate the range of motion of a body part (e.g., Hip Moves).

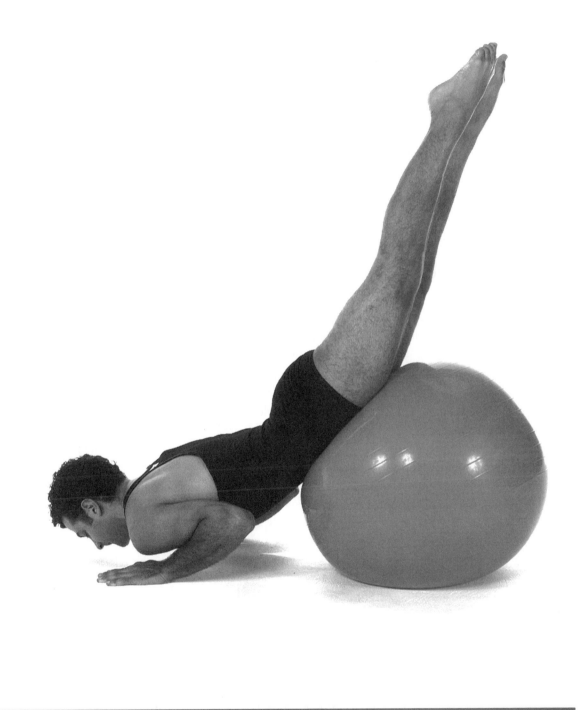

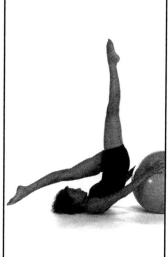

eight principles of Pilates

Joseph Pilates' book, *Return to Life*, maps out the eight important principles that underlie the Pilates method. When Pilates exercises are done with the following concepts in mind, you will gain much more meaning and effectiveness in your workout.

Control

As I mentioned earlier, Joseph Pilates originally called his method "Contrology" (it wasn't until his students began teaching for him that people started referring to the method as Pilates). One of the fundamental rules when doing Pilates: Control your body's every movement! This rule applies not only to the exercises themselves but also to transitions between exercises, how you get on and off the equipment, and your overall attention to detail while working out. When doing mat exercises, control comes into play with the attack and ending of each movement. When the body puts on the brakes in a controlled manner, it is training the muscles to work as they lengthen. This is called eccentric muscle contraction, which builds long and flexible muscles. Also, when focusing on control of a movement, the body is forced to recruit helper muscles (we call these synergists), which are usually smaller than the main muscles. When many muscles work together to do one movement, or when muscles work synergistically, the body as a whole develops greater balance and coordination. Also, the big muscles won't get too big and bulky because they don't have to do all the work by themselves. Thus we become a long and lean machine. Once your body learns to move with control you will feel more confident doing all kinds of things from hiking a rocky cliff, to salsa dancing, or to standing on a chair to reach an out-of-the-way martini glass.

Breath

I have heard that most people use something like 50 percent of their lung capacity when they breathe. Shallow breathing is an unfortunate side effect of a sedentary and stressful life. Moreover, people actually hold their breath when performing a new or difficult task. When training Pilates clients, I have to tell them to exhale, or else often they won't! When you hold your breath, you tense muscles that can ultimately exacerbate improper posture and reinforce tension habits. That is why consistent breathing is essential to flowing movement and proper muscle balance. As with yoga,

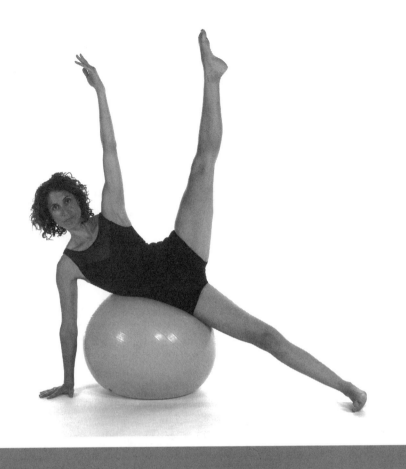

breathing is an essential part of the Pilates method and distinguishes it from other exercise forms.

Every Pilates exercise has a specific breathing pattern assigned to it. Breathing while moving is not always an easy assignment, but when accomplished, beautiful things can happen. Focused breath can help maximize the body's ability to stretch, and through this release of tension you will gain optimal body control. Deep inhalation and full exhalation also exercises the lungs and increases lung capacity, bringing deep relaxation as a pleasant side effect.

Flowing Movement

Many of the moves in Pilates look a lot like yoga. But unlike yoga, we do not hold positions—instead we flow from movement to movement. In this way Pilates is more like dance, in that the flow of the body is essential to doing Pilates correctly. When doing a Pilates workout, you want to flow and move freely during the movement phase and finish with control and precision. This way of moving brings flexibility to the joints and muscles while training the body to elongate and move with an even rhythm. Flowing movement integrates the nervous system,

the muscles, and the joints, and trains the body to move smoothly and evenly.

Precision

Precision is a lot like control but has the added element of spatial awareness. When attacking any movement you must know exactly where that movement starts and ends. All Pilates exercises have precise definitions of where the body should be at all times: the angle of the legs, the placement of the elbows, the positioning of the head and neck, even what the fingers are doing! The little things count in Pilates. This kind of precision in movement will resonate in the rest of your life. If you suffer from pain because of faulty postural habits that you aren't even aware of, after a few good sessions with a competent Pilates instructor you will be pleasantly surprised by how fast a new-found awareness can affect a positive change in your body. This change can only happen when you begin to notice your physical habits and increase the precision in your movements.

Centering

Sometimes we joke at my studio that we should have subliminal tapes running all day that say "Pull the navel to the spine." Why? Because this is the mantra of any worthy Pilates trainer. All exercises are done with the deep abdominals engaged to ensure proper centering. Most Pilates exercises focus on developing abdominal strength either directly or indirectly. Never forget to pull in the belly or you will be reprimanded by the Pilates Goddess! Even when performing an exercise that focuses on strengthening the arm muscles, you should keep your abdominal scoop, keep your shoulders pulling down the back, and perhaps even squeeze your butt. All these actions promote centering and core muscle strength. No exercise should be done to the detriment of center control. In other words, if your center is not totally and completely engaged and

stabilized, you may not progress to the next level of an exercise.

Stability

Ever wonder what makes Pilates such an excellent back rehabilitation method? The lion's share of Pilates exercises utilize the concept of torso stability, which is key to the health and longevity of your spine. Now what is stability? Basically, it is the ability to *not* move a part of the body while another part is challenging it. Maintaining stillness in the spine as you move the arms and legs requires torso stability, accomplished mainly by the abdominal muscles. After an injury, there is generally instability in the affected area. The first thing you want to do is learn to stabilize the injured part so as to prevent re-injury and to allow the healing process to begin. Thus, Pilates is one of the safest forms of exercise to do after injury. Pilates will also prevent injury, for if you have excellent stability in your torso and joints, you are much less likely to injure yourself in the first place.

Range of Motion

"Range of motion" is a phrase used by medical professionals to describe how much movement a part of the body can perform. For instance, the range of motion of your shoulder joint is defined by how high you can raise your arm in front of you, behind you, etc. Your range of motion

can be affected by your muscles, bones, and other tissues such as ligaments and fascia (connective tissue). Basically, range of motion is just another way of describing flexibility. Pilates exercises are meant to increase the range of motion of your spine or joints if you are too tight. If you are too flexible (yes, this is possible!) then Pilates exercises will help you to learn the proper range of motion for your spine or joints. It is important to understand how to limit your range of motion if you lack stability because this will help to prevent injury in the future.

Opposition

In any great story there is a protagonist and an antagonist, the hero and the bad guy. Similarly, for each muscle in your body there is an opposing muscle that performs an opposite movement. These are called agonists and antagonists. If the agonist is tight, the antagonist will be weak or will be unable to contract fully. This is an essential concept to grasp when conditioning your body. If you wonder why it's so hard for you to straighten your legs in front of you when sitting up, it's because your hamstrings are tight. Your quadriceps are the muscles that straighten your legs, but if your hamstrings are super-tight, then the quads have to work overtime to straighten the legs.

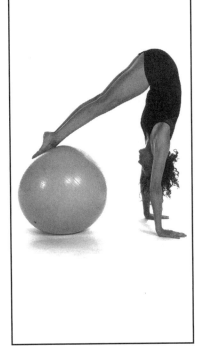

general movement vocabulary

Articulation

This is another word for range of motion. We use this word mainly when referring to moving the spine one vertebra at a time while rounding down the mat, as opposed to coming down in one piece.

Parallel vs. Turn-out

If you've ever taken a modern dance class then you probably have heard the terms parallel legs and turned-out legs. Simply put, parallel means your legs are neutral, with knees facing forward—as most of us do naturally when we stand. Turn-out or external rotation of the hips means your knees and feet are facing away from each other and your leg bones are laterally rotated in the hip socket. All ballet dance is done in turn-out, while modern dance often has movements that use the legs in parallel. In Pilates, we do many exercises in turn-out (see Pilates "V" from the Pilates Alphabet above). Why turn-out? Because it engages both the butt and inner thighs, and can help stabilize your pelvis during certain exercises.

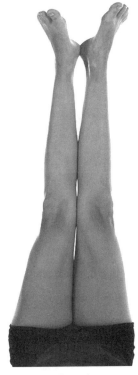
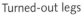

Turned-out legs

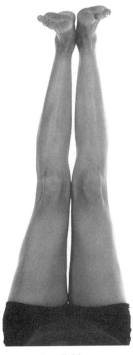

Parallel legs

Supine

This is a term that simply means lying on your back. Think spine (supine with the "u" taken out).

Prone

This term means lying on your belly.

The Powerhouse

The Powerhouse is a term that came from Joe Pilates himself, used today mostly by New York trainers. The abdominals, butt, and inner thigh muscles, when working together, constitute the Powerhouse. This is where many of the Pilates exercises can be initiated. It is also the area that is challenged in many exercises. These muscles are the main stabilizing muscles of the body and are very important for preventing injury to the spine.

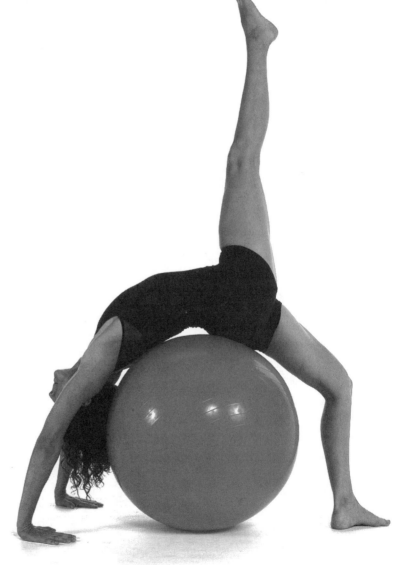

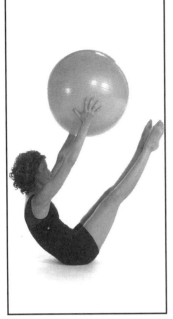

Ellie Herman's Pilates alphabet

Just as every word can be broken down into letters, so can every Pilates exercise be broken down into discrete parts. The Pilates alphabet is my way to facilitate the learning process and demystify even the most complex Pilates exercises. Almost every advanced exercise contains basic movements that repeat over and over in the repertoire.

Abdominal Scoop

The Abdominal Scoop can be done anywhere and at any time, and frankly it should be done as much as possible. Pulling the navel in toward the spine, thinking of zipping up a tight pair of pants, or sucking in your spare tire will all do the job. What you are doing anatomically is engaging your deepest abdominal muscles, which function to hold in your viscera and, when contracted, decrease the diameter of the abdominal wall. The Abdominal Scoop works a lot like a drawstring around a pair of sweat pants when pulled taut. You have four layers of abdominal muscles; your deepest one is called the *transversus abdominis*. The second and third layers are called your *internal* and *external* obliques. And the most superficial abdominal layer is called your rectus abdominis. The rectus (as we Pilates instructors call it) is a workaholic muscle and will do all the work if you let it. The Abdominal

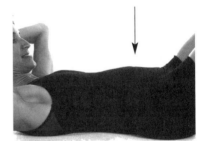

Here I'm pooching:
No pooching allowed!

Scoop, or "navel to spine" image is meant to bring in the deeper three layers, which work to compress the abdominal wall and help support the back. In every exercise you want to be using your Abdominal Scoop to get the most profound results possible. Pooching is the opposite of scooping—No pooching allowed!

Here I'm scooping

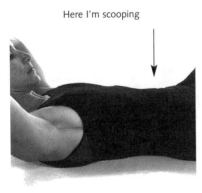

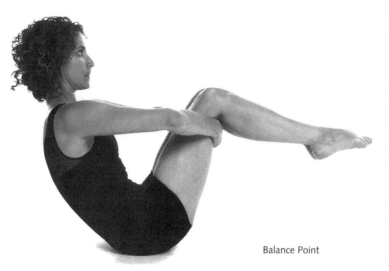

Balance Point

Balance Point

Balance Point is a position in which you begin and end the rolling exercises in the Pilates mat repertoire; it is also the place you arrive at the top of the Teaser. You can practice Balance Point by sitting up with your knees bent, holding on to the backs of your thighs. Roll back slightly behind your tailbone, pull your belly in, and lift your feet off the floor. In order to maintain your balance and stop yourself from rolling backward, you must engage and pull in your deep abdominal muscles and slightly round the low back. This teaches you that to balance with ease, you must engage your deep abdominals.

Bridge

Bridge is a basic position in Pilates as well as a beginning-level exercise on the mat and the ball. In kinesiological terms, a bridge is extension of the hips. In lay terms, this means lifting your hips up off the floor, using your butt and hamstrings to do

so. It's part of the Pilates Alphabet because it is a position we come in and out of during various exercises. I want to point out that a bridge should be done from the hip extensors (butt and

hamstrings) and not from the back muscles. Therefore when doing a bridge you must keep your spine neutral and make sure not to arch the back!

C-Curve

Martha Graham was the first person to introduce the idea of C-curve into modern dance. Before Graham, dancers performed ballet or used the Isadora Duncan technique, which has the spine always erect, extended, elegant, and otherworldly. Graham introduced spinal flexion, or what she termed "the contraction," which revolutionized dance. It was a primal, dark, and oh-so-human

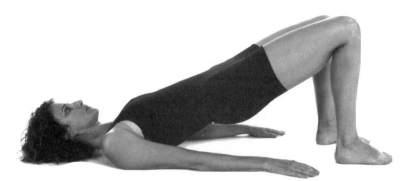

Correct Bridge: The back is neutral

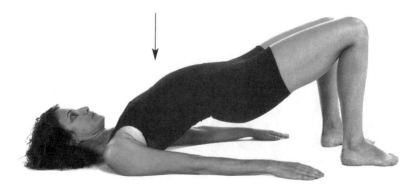

Incorrect Bridge: The back is hyperextended

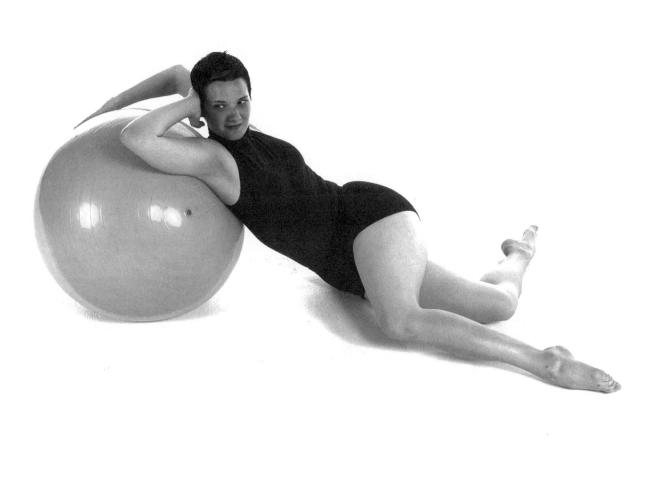

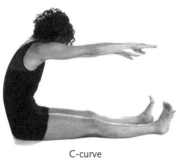

C-curve

movement. It put us back onto the earth from some other world. Joe Pilates worked with Graham in his Eighth Avenue studio and learned a couple of tricks from her. The C-curve is rounding of the back, or flexion of the spine. The "C" is meant to describe the shape of the back after you scoop in your belly. This shape should always be initiated by your deep abdominal scoop and should provide a lovely stretch for your spine. Many Pilates exercises use the C-curve.

Door Frame Arms

Arms are straight in front of you, shoulder distance apart, making the shape of the outer frame of a door. This describes the shape of your arms in many Pilates exercises, whether your arms are above your head, by your sides when lying supine on the

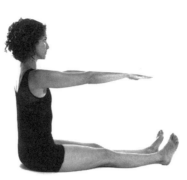

Door Frame Arms

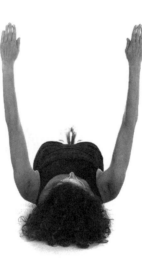

Door Frame Arms

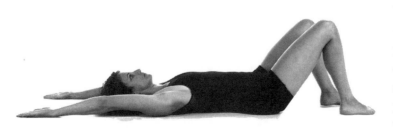

Door Frame Arms

floor, or supporting you in a plank position.

Hip-Up

The name says it all. Lie on your back with your legs up, your knees bent, and your Door Frame Arms down by your sides. Rock back and lift your hips up by using your low Abdominal Scoop. The Hip-up works your lower abdominals and can be very challenging for those with a weak tummy, a tight back, or a large butt!

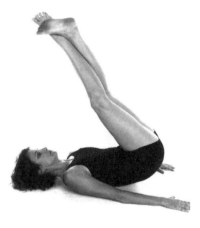

Hip-up

Levitation

When you combine a Hip-up with a little low butt squeeze, you get Levitation. What the low butt squeeze is actually doing is extending the hip. In kinesiological terms, a Hip-up by itself is merely the flexion of the spine, but when you squeeze your butt, you add an extension of the hips—put them together and you have Levitation. Try it if you like: lie on your back, lift up your hips with your Abdominal Scoop, and at the top of the Hip-

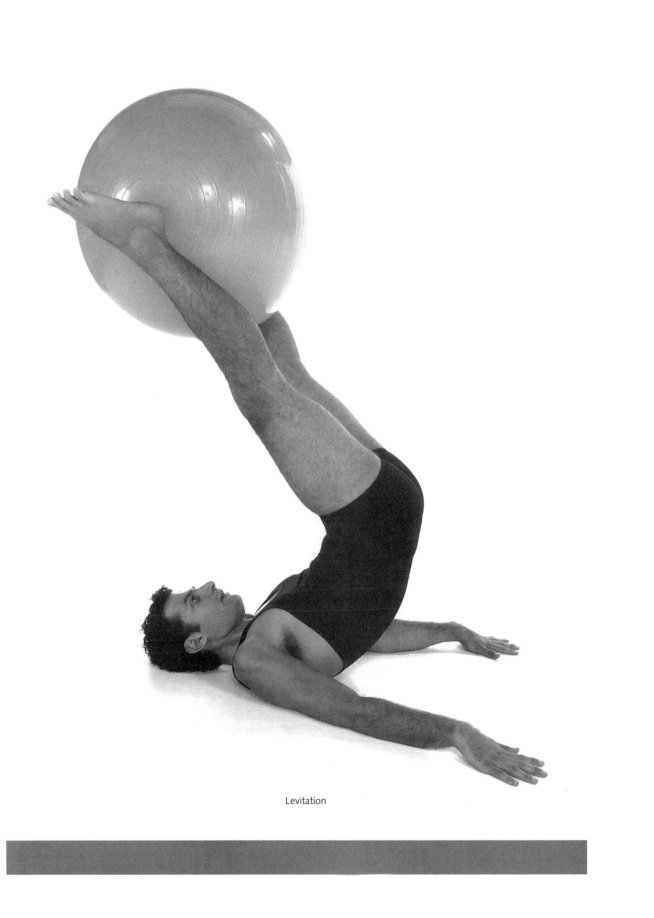

Levitation

up, squeeze your butt. You'll feel your hips levitate, rising perceptibly higher, as if the hand of Houdini came down and lifted your hips magically and effortlessly off the floor.

Neutral Spine

If you've ever wondered what the heck the difference is between the New York and the West Coast Pilates schools, I've got two words for you: Neutral Spine. Neutral Spine is one of the most subtle yet powerful principles in Ellie Herman's Pilates Alphabet. Like much of Pilates, understanding Neutral Spine requires an understanding of your body and anatomy. Neutral Spine can be felt when lying down on your back, knees bent and feet flat on the floor. Your spine should have two areas that do not touch the floor beneath you: your neck and your low back (cervical and lumbar spine, respectively). One way to visualize Neutral Spine is to imagine you have a pitcher of

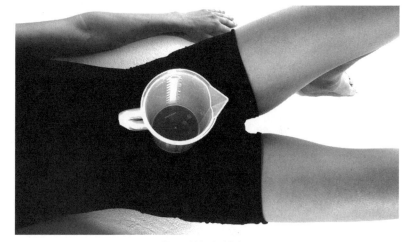

Correct Neutral Spine

hot water balanced on your low belly. When you are in neutral, your pitcher should not spill and should be perfectly balanced. If your pelvis is tilted forward (arching your low back too much off the floor) or tilted posteriorly (flattening your low back onto the floor), your pitcher will spill in one of those directions. Your tailbone should be grounded onto the floor.

To get technical: Neutral pelvis is actually defined as the pubic bone and the hip bones (*anterior superior iliac spine*, or

the asis for short) being on the same plane. You can feel these bony landmarks with your fingers when you're lying down, and this triangle of bones, when neutral, should create a flat table for your pitcher. The reason we care about Neutral Spine is that this is the healthiest position for your spine when standing up—when your spine is neutral you have natural curves. These curves function to absorb shock when running, jumping, or simply walking around town. And ultimately if you live in Neutral Spine, you will be putting the least amount of stress on the muscles and bones. That's the beauty of perfect posture: it actually feels better. We want to maintain and reinforce these natural curves and that is why we often work in Neutral Spine when performing stability exercises in Pilates. Many people from the New York school teach people to "tuck under" or flatten the curve of their low back when doing Pilates exercises or when

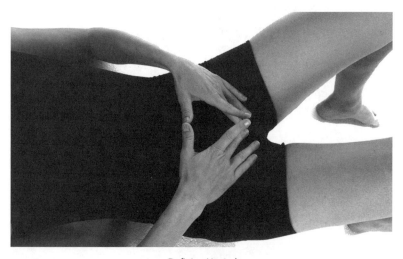

Defining Neutral

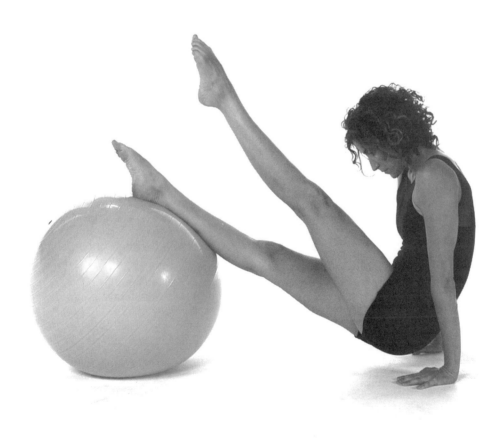

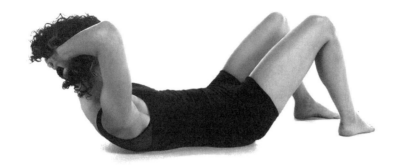

Pilates Abdominal Positioning

neck and you will not be using your abdominals as much. The upper abdominals should be working to maintain this position (and that's where you should feel the burn).

Pilates "V" (Pilates First Position)

If you've ever taken a dance class, you probably know that First Position means standing with your legs together and turned out from the hip, knees facing away from each other, and feet making a V shape. The Pilates V is very much the same except you never want to force the turn-out. Your feet should be making a V shape, but I always say this V should be the shape of a slice of pie, not a huge slice but a nice small Pilates-size

standing. This method is no longer thought to be posturally correct; instead, the natural curve or Neutral Spine is preferred.

Pilates Abdominal Positioning

The Pilates Abdominal Position-ing is my way to describe the placement of the upper body when performing many of the supine Pilates floor exercises. When lying on your back (supine), lift your head off the floor just high enough so that the bottom tips of your shoulder blades are either just touching or just off the floor. Imagine that the base of the sternum is anchored to the floor and the back of the neck and upper back are stretching around that anchor. Make sure to keep a space the size of a tangerine under your chin (see below); you are not meant to over-stretch the back of your neck.

It is essential to maintain this position when performing abdominal exercises. If you allow the head to drop back you will begin to feel fatigue in the

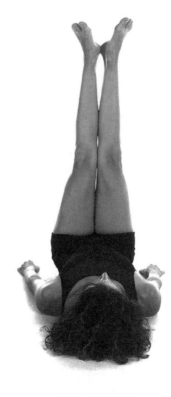

Pilates First Position

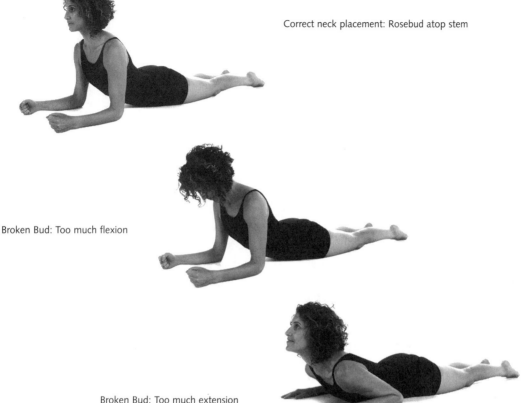

Correct neck placement: Rosebud atop stem

Broken Bud: Too much flexion

Broken Bud: Too much extension

slice. In Pilates, instead of keeping your legs parallel, we use this First Position in many exercises. Why? Because externally rotating the hips engages the gluteus maximus and the inner thigh muscles, which we like to use as much as possible in Pilates. (See Parallel vs. Turn-out, above.)

Rosebud

Have you ever gotten a bunch of roses and one of them has a broken bud? You know, one bud that droops down sadly, almost detached from its stem. If you imagine your head as the bud and your spine as the stem in a healthy unbroken rose, then in

any movement your spine makes the bud will follow and continue the curve of the spine in a smooth line. When you move your head in a "faulty" sequence (say, when you come up into a Swan or perform back extension from lying on your belly), your head can look like a broken bud; that is, your neck is bent at a greater angle than the rest of your spine. We want no broken buds in Pilates! Only healthy, happy roses and spines.

Squeeze a Tangerine

This is an image that describes the sequencing of your head as you lift it off the floor. It also shows the distance your chin

should be from your chest when holding your Pilates Abdominal positioning. The size of a tangerine is precisely the amount of space that should be between your chin and your chest when doing a spinal flexion.

Stacking the Spine

Stacking the Spine is a finish to several exercises in the Pilates method. Stacking the Spine teaches spinal articulation as well as how to sit up vertically. It is a way to sit up or stand erect from a hunched-over position. Stacking the Spine begins with the lowest part of the spine and stacks up, one vertebra at a time, the head staying heavy and

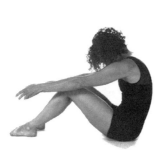

Stacking the Spine 1

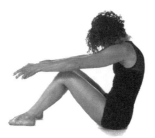

Stacking the Spine 2

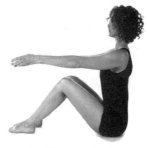

Stacking the Spine 3

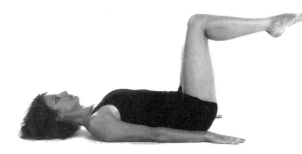

Table Top Legs

Torso stability

Torso stability is accomplished mainly by abdominal strength and is one of the most important concepts in the Pilates method. Most Pilates exercises require you to maintain a stable torso while the arms or legs move. Again, the abdominals are responsible for keeping the spine still while forces are moving around it. So when you are doing one of these stability exercises (and you can tell if it is a stability exercise if you hold the torso in one place for the duration of the exercise), simply think to yourself, "Don't move." This is the essence of stability.

dropped until the very end. The spine should be completely vertical at the end, with the natural curves of the back in place. (This can be practiced against a wall to better feel the vertical alignment of the spine.)

Table Top Legs

Table Top Legs describes the position of your legs when you are lying supine (on your back), with the knees and feet up off the floor, inner thighs pulling to-gether, knees bent at a 90-degree angle, and the thighs at a 90-degree angle to the floor.

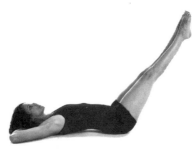

Poor Torso Stability:
Incorrect placement of the spine

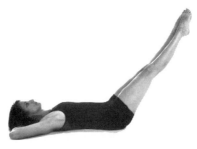

Strong Torso Stability: Correct placement
of the spine—abdominals
keep back flat on floor

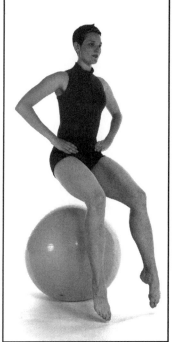

how to use this book

This book is structured like a ball class. If you are healthy and you simply crave full body conditioning, you can follow the workout in the order it is presented in the book. But whatever you do, don't skip the Trouble-shooting section, especially if you suffer from chronic pain or injury.

The Levels

Do the beginning exercises until you feel comfortable with the concepts and the movements. Then add the intermediate exercises, and after a few months of conditioning, you can try the advanced and super-advanced exercises. Remember, the levels of the exercises are meant to help you learn the Pilates method in a natural progression for your body. Most importantly, the levels are meant to help you not hurt yourself. The intermediate and advanced exercises require a fair amount of core strength to perform properly. You could injure your back if you try to push yourself beyond your level. Please read the Dos and Don'ts for each exercise carefully to make sure you are performing the exercise with the correct form. If you feel strain in your low back or neck at anytime, please do not continue with the movement, but look for modifications instead.

The Order

- Begin with the bouncing aerobic warm-up. If you don't like bouncing because it makes you dizzy or gives you a headache, skip it.
- Continue your warm-up with a series of Hip Moves to open up your low back and hips.
- Then begin the Essential Workout, a series that follows a close-to-classic Pilates mat repertoire. (There are a few reformer-based exercises thrown into the Essential Workout section.)
- The Essential Workout also contains several targeted series built around specific moves, such as Plank, Bridge, and Roll-downs. These increase the challenge for particular body pars, including arms, abs, and butt.
- Finish your workout with a series of cool downs and lovely stretches for your spine and hips.

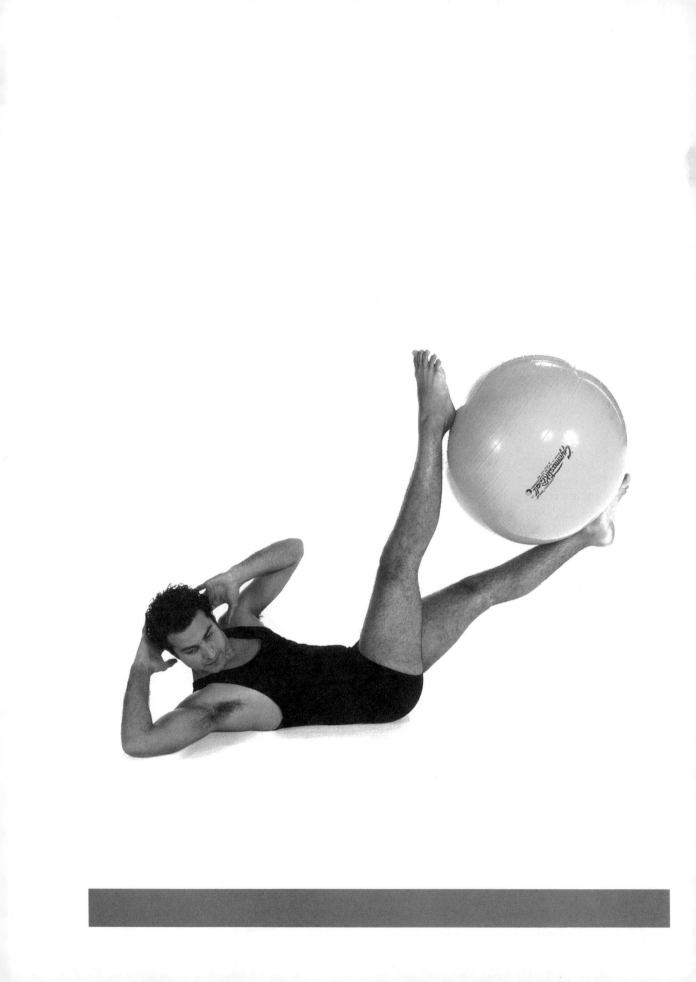

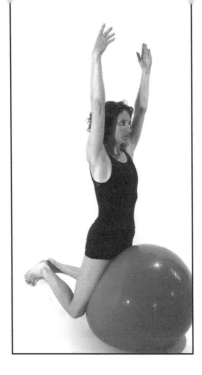

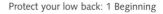

Trouble-shooting, or, Do Not Skip This Section

When learning new exercises it is common for certain aches and pains to develop. The following are a few common problems that people face when they are still in the process of gaining strength and stability. Please read through this section even if you don't have any of these problems yet. The point is to prevent potential overuse or strain of your muscles and tissues.

How to modify to protect your low back

In general if you suffer from low back pain you need to know a few tips to keep you from further contributing to your problems. Always modify any exercise that requires you to support your legs out in front of you while keeping your belly scooped or your back flat on the mat. Experiment with the following modifications:

- Don't use a ball if the exercise requires you to hold it between your legs.

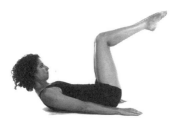
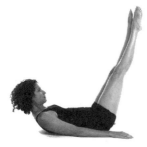

Protect your low back: 1 Beginning   2 Intermediate   3 Advanced

- Bend your knees if the exercise requires straight legs.
- Keep your legs high enough so that you can absolutely maintain a scooped belly and a flat back on the mat.
- Stop if you feel back strain and do a psoas stretch. In fact, you should do a Psoas Stretch everyday after you warm up (see page 110).

How to avoid wrist compression when up on your arms

- Spread your fingers and press into all of them when weight-bearing. Focus especially on pressing into the thumb, forefinger, and pinky.
- Try to "cup" your wrist when weight-bearing. That is, lift up the middle of your palm to

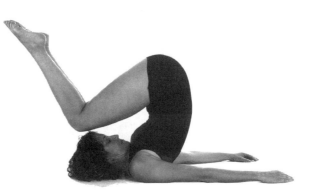

Incorrect neck placement:
Don't roll onto your neck

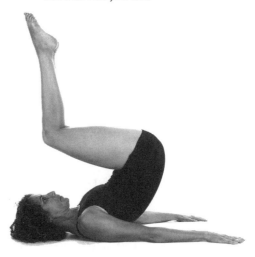

Correct neck placement:
Balance between shoulder blades

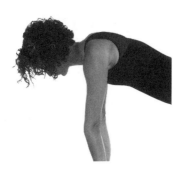

Incorrect: Avoid dropping into wrists, elbows and shoulders

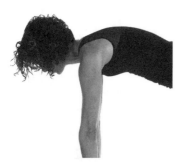

Correct: Lift up from the wrists and shoulders and soften the elbows

decrease putting weight into your wrist joint proper.

- Keep your shoulders properly aligned. Think of rolling the shoulder blades down away from the ears so you are supporting your body weight from the back muscles.
- Think of pressing away from the ground with your back strength.
- Don't let your weight bear down into the wrist; instead, press away from gravity.
- Don't hyperextend elbows: keep the inner elbow ceases facing each other.

How to do a rolling exercise: Never onto your neck!

There are several exercises on the floor in which you are required to roll onto your upper back. (Rolling Like a Ball, Open Leg Rocker, Rollover, etc.).

- Do not roll onto your neck; instead, stop and balance between your shoulder blades.
- Use control when rolling back. Don't roll back so fast that you can't control your momentum.
- Scoop your abdominals in to help stop yourself from rolling back too far.

What size ball is right for you and ball maintenance:

What size ball should you buy? Well, my basic rule is that when sitting on the ball, you should be able to easily balance with your feet on the ground. Your hips and knees should both be at right angles. If the ball is too big, it will feel like you are rolling forward off the ball. If the ball is too small, your hips will be at less than a right angle and you'll feel like you can't really sit up tall. The following list details the right size ball for you:

- 55 centimeter if you are under 5'
- 65 centimeter for 5'-5'7"
- 75 centimeter if you are 5'8"-6'2"
- 1.85 centimeter if you are over 6'2"

You can vary the size and squishiness of the ball by how much air you put in it. If blown very taut, the ball will be bigger and more difficult to balance on. Ideally, the ball should have a little rebound when pushed—but not so much that it feels soggy. My friend carol actually blew up her physioball with her mouth, but I would recommend a bicycle pump, a foot pump, or for the fastest blow up, the air-pump at a gas station.

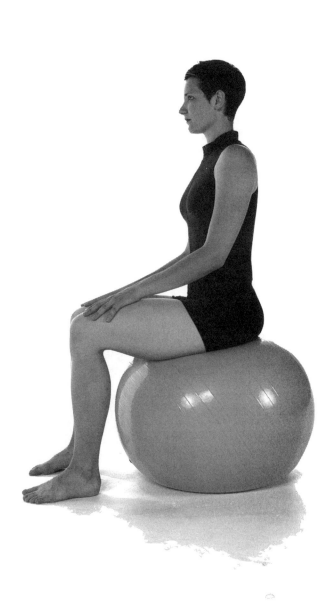

Correct ball size

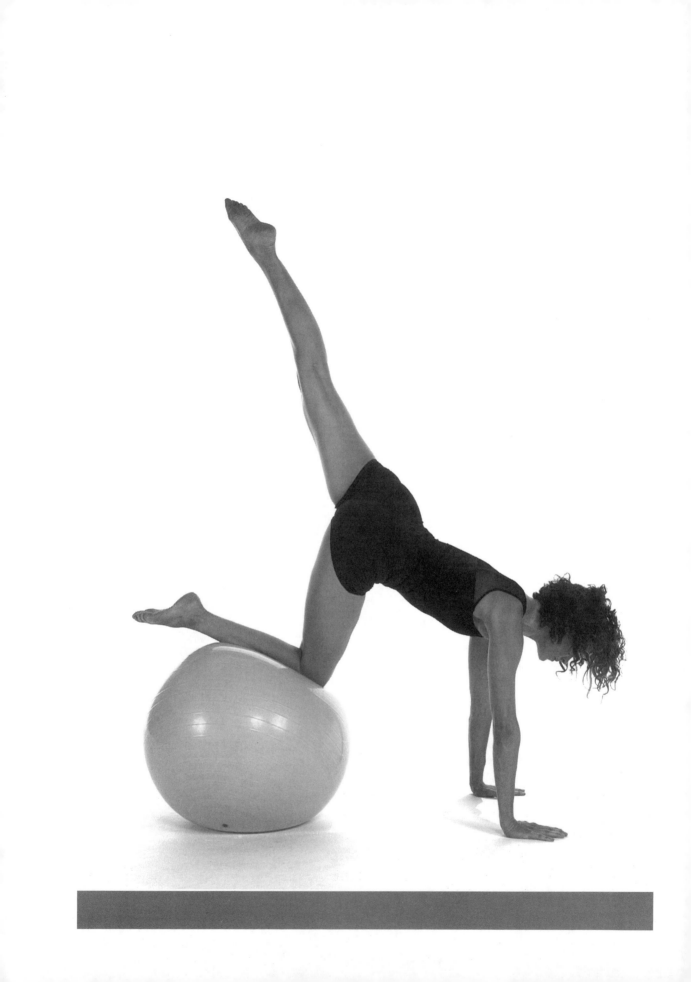

part one:

aerobic

warm-up

basic bouncing
beginning

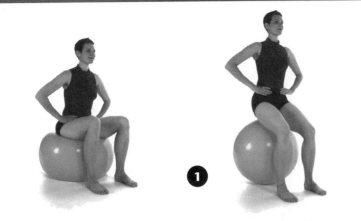

STARTING POSITION: Sit on the ball, legs a little wider than hip distance apart, hands on hips. Feet face front, with knees, hips, and feet in line.

1 Breathe continuously. Bounce up and down, keeping your feet firmly planted on the floor.

repeat 8–32 times

clapping above your head
beginning

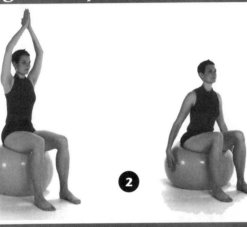

1 Continue bouncing. At the top of your bounce, clap your hands.

2 At the bottom of your bounce, hit the ball.

repeat 8–32 times

chicken wings
beginning

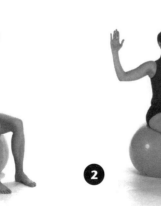

1 Continue bouncing. At the top of your bounce, clap your hands.

2 As you descend, bend your elbows to a 90-degree angle and think of pulling them down behind your body. This is a stretch for your chest and a strengthening exercise for your back.

repeat 8–32 times

DOS & DON'TS FOR BOUNCING SERIES

- Don't wear socks—you might slip. Do this in either bare feet or sneakers.
- Scoop your belly in every time you go up, as if you were lifting up from your center.
- Keep your head in line with your hips. Don't let your head lead forward or back, because this will take your bounce off center.
- Keep your shoulders relaxed and down.

IMAGINE

- You are gleefully doing the hippity-hop.

bouncing series

drumming
intermediate

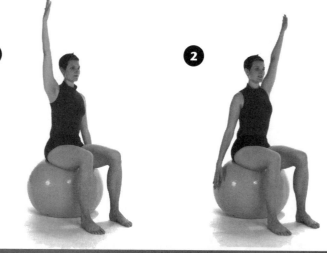

1 Continue bouncing. Lift one arm up at the top of the bounce as the other hits the ball.

2 Alternate arms continually, creating an even drumming rhythm as you bounce.

repeat 8–32 times

kick forward
intermediate

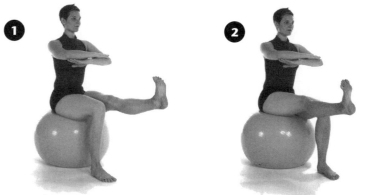

1 Continue bouncing. Fold your arms in front of your chest (a la "I Dream of Jeannie"). Feet face front, with knees, hips, and feet in line. Start to bounce, then try to lift one leg off and kick it forward for one bounce before replacing it.

2 Alternate legs.

repeat 8–16 times

cossack
intermediate

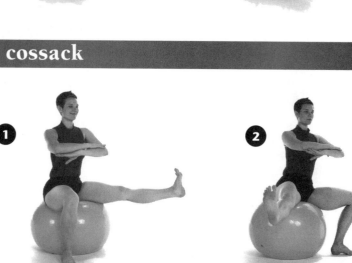

1 Open your legs and turn them out. Kick one leg out to the side as you bear most of your weight on the bent leg on the floor. Lean toward the weight-bearing leg, so you will be rocking from side to side.

2 Alternate legs. This can be done slowly at first without bouncing, then when you get the hang of it try to get some air time.

repeat 8–16 times

jumping in parallel   *intermediate*

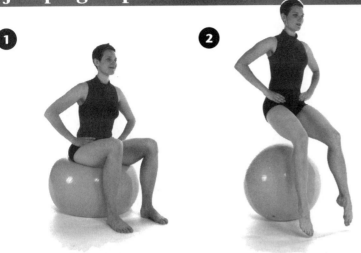

1–2 Instead of keeping your feet planted, push through your feet and jump off the floor, pointing your toes in the air. Keep your legs in parallel, with feet, knees, and hips in alignment. Always keep your weight slightly forward when bouncing. Don't ever land on the ball with your weight back or you risk flying backward onto your head.

repeat   8 times

jumping in turn-out   *intermediate*

1 Open your legs wide in turn-out, making sure to keep your knees aiming over your middle toes. Push through your feet and jump off the floor, pointing your feet in the air.

repeat   8 times

exploding star   *intermediate*

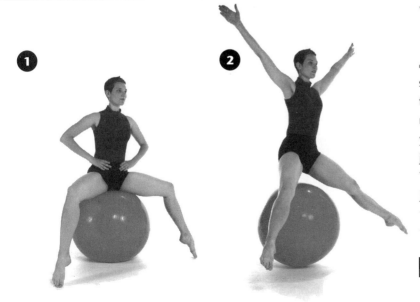

1 Start with Jumping In Turn-out.

2 At the height of your jump, extend your arms and legs like a star in four directions. This is one of the most aerobic exercises in the series because it takes work to keep your arms stretched, as well as to jump explosively with your legs. You should travel forward on each jump. Don't ever land on the ball with your weight back or you risk flying backward onto your head.

repeat   8 times

bouncing series

hop around the ball

intermediate

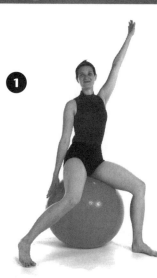

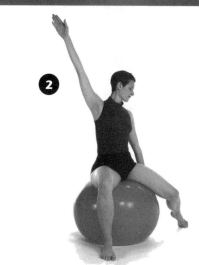

1–6 Using Drumming Arms, allow your legs to lightly jump your feet from side to side. The trick is to not let the feet bear too much weight; keep it light. Keeping a rhythm, travel in one direction, making a full circle. It should take 8-10 jumps to complete a full rotation. Then reverse directions.

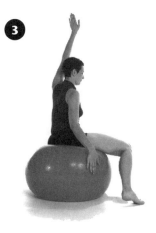

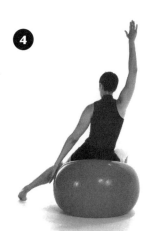

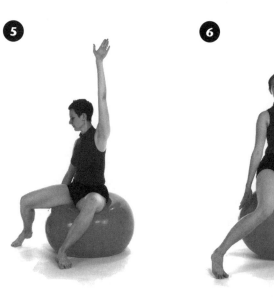

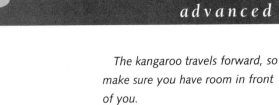

1

2

3

The kangaroo travels forward, so make sure you have room in front of you.

1–3 Keep your legs in parallel, and as you go up in your jump, pull the ball forward with your tailbone, using your Abdominal Scoop. You should travel forward on every bounce. Make sure when you land back on the ball you have neutral pelvis or else you will be catapulted forward. Also, remember to always land on the center of the ball, not too far back or your weight will fly back with you.

repeat **8 times**

Ellie's bouncing recipe

It's fun to make up a long routine combining different jumps. Adding an aerobic component to your workout is important for weight loss and the general health of the lungs and heart. Put on your favorite dance music—preferably with a good bouncing beat. Repeat until you've done 15 minutes of bouncing!

Here's one idea:
8 bounces with hands on hips.
8 bounces with Clapping.
8 bounces with Chicken Wings.
8 Kick Forward into 8 Cossack into 8 Kick Forward.
8 bounces with Drumming.

Hopping Around the Ball in a circle.
8 Kangaroos followed by Hopping Around the Ball halfway, 8 Kangaroos back, then hop around back to front.
8 Jumping in Parallels.
8 Jumping In Turn-outs.
8 Exploding Stars.

side-to-side
intermediate

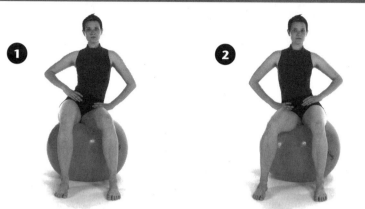

STARTING POSITION: Sit up on top of the ball with your hands on your hips, feet placed on the floor a little wider than hip distance apart.

1–2 Breathe continuously. Rock your hips from side to side.

repeat 8 times

front and back
intermediate

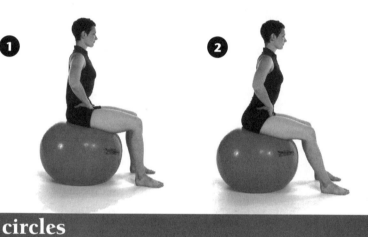

1 Rock your hips forward. Think of initiating the movement from your belly, scooping in and creating a C-curve.

2 Rock your hips back, thinking of sticking your butt out and arching your back.

repeat 8 times

circles
intermediate

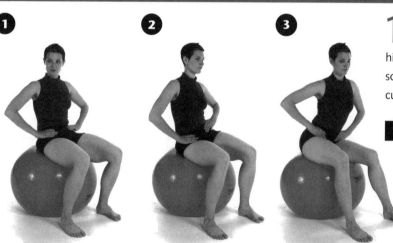

1–3 Inscribe the biggest circle you can with your hips. As you come to the front, scoop your belly in and make a C-curve with your lower back.

repeat 8 times

BENEFITS OF HIP MOVES
- Loosens the hips and low back.
- It's fun.

DOS & DON'TS
- Do keep the ball centered underneath your pelvis; don't let it get out of control.
- Do feel the abdominals controlling the movement of the ball forward.

part two:
essential
workout

breathing in neutral spine

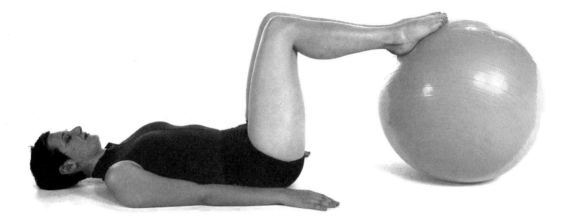

STARTING POSITION: Lie on your back with your legs relaxed up on the ball, knees bent. Your back should be relaxed on the floor, in Neutral Spine. **INHALE TO BEGIN.**

1 As you breathe in, expand fully into your back and laterally into your ribcage, like an expanding accordion. Try not to let your belly pooch out as you inhale.

2 **EXHALE:** Slowly allow the breath to leave your lungs, letting your abdominal muscles drop down into your back like layers of blankets settling in the wind.

repeat **3 times**

BENEFITS	DOS & DON'TS	IMAGINE
■ Gets you in touch with your deep abdominals, especially your transversus abdominis. ■ Teaches how to breathe fully. ■ Allows you to feel and understand Neutral Spine.	■ Keep Neutral Spine—i.e., pubic bone and hip bones create a plane parallel to the floor. ■ Don't tuck your pelvis or flatten your lower back.	■ A tea cup full of tea is balanced on your low belly. If your pelvis rocks forward or back, you will spill the tea and also come out of Neutral Spine.

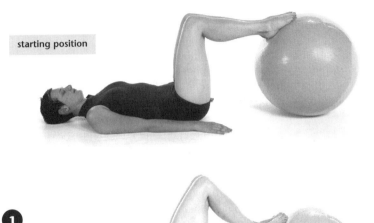

starting position

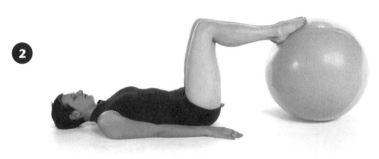

1

2

STARTING POSITION: Lie on your back, knees bent and feet on the ball. **INHALE TO BEGIN**.

1 **EXHALE:** Pull the navel in toward your spine and flatten your back onto the floor, slowly rolling your tailbone upward, one vertebra at a time. **INHALE:** Hold.

2 **EXHALE:** Retrograde the movement by rolling down one vertebra at a time, going through the flat back until you arrive finally in Neutral Spine. **INHALE** and repeat.

| repeat | 3 times |

BENEFITS

- Puts you in touch with your deep abdominals, especially your transversus abdominis.
- Teaches how the abdominals move the spine.
- Creates articulation, movement, and stretch in the low back.
- Shows the difference between Neutral Spine and flat back.

DOS & DON'TS

- Initiate the movement of your spine from your abdominals, not your butt! You could perform this same movement from the gluteals, but that is not the goal of this exercise.

- Don't come up so high that your back is extended (arched). If you feel your neck, you've gone too high. Keep your butt fairly low to the floor.
- Make sure you go through the flat back on the way up and the way down from the curl. This is how you really feel the deep Abdominal Scoop!
- If you have a very tight low back it may be difficult for you to find the flat back. But this is a great way to get some movement in that area.
- If you have overdeveloped abdominals (especially the superficial rectus abdominis) you will find that pulling the belly in is quite a challenge. Remember, don't push out—pull the belly in!

IMAGINE

- As you pull in your belly to flatten your back on the floor, you are creating an imprint with your spine on an imaginary sandy beach beneath your back. We call this "imprinting" in the Pilates world.

upper abdominal curls

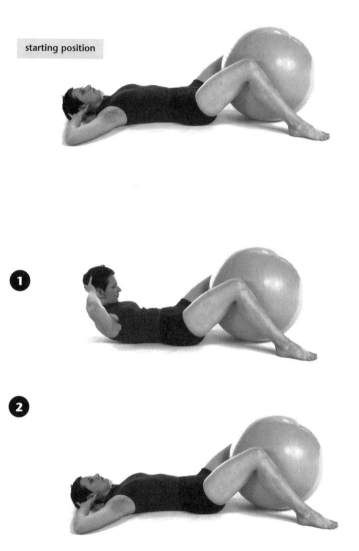

starting position

1

2

STARTING POSITION: Lie on your back with your hands interlaced behind your head. Your ball is between your legs. Keep it there by gently squeezing your inner thighs. **INHALE TO BEGIN**.

1 **EXHALE:** Squeeze the ball firmly between your thighs and scoop your belly in as you Squeeze a Tangerine under your chin to lift your head off the floor. Keep curling up until your shoulder blades are just off the floor or until you are in what I call the Pilates Abdominal Positioning.

2 **INHALE:** Retrograde the movement with control.

| repeat | 8 times |

BENEFITS	DOS & DON'TS
■ Strengthens neck flexors, abdominals, and inner thighs.	■ Keep your Abdominal Scoop the whole time.
■ Shows how to keep neutral pelvis while flexing the neck and upper back.	■ Make sure you Squeeze a Tangerine to ensure proper sequencing of the neck.
■ Teaches how to keep your Abdominal Scoop while curling up.	■ Maintain Neutral Spine throughout the exercise; don't let your pelvis tuck under.
	■ Look at your belly as you roll up to make sure you're not pooching out.
	■ Don't do if you have an acute neck injury or if it feels bad on your neck.

first position
beginning

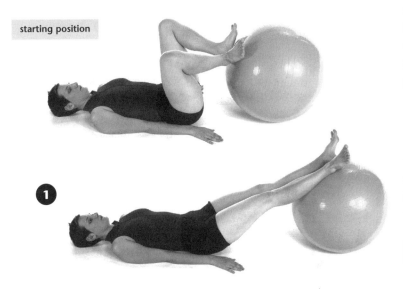

starting position

STARTING POSITION: Lie on your back, knees bent, and put your feet turned out on top of the ball, knees open in Pilates First Position. **INHALE TO BEGIN**.

1 EXHALE: Extend your legs away from you, pulling the inner thighs together as you straighten the legs completely. **INHALE** to return to starting position and repeat.

| repeat | 10 times |

heels in parallel
beginning

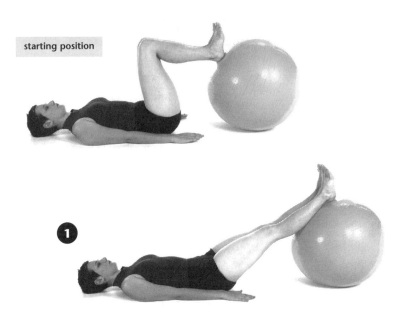

starting position

STARTING POSITION: Begin with your knees and ankles squeezing together, feet flexed on top of the ball. **INHALE TO BEGIN.**

1 EXHALE: Gently press your heels downward onto the ball as you extend your legs straight out, making sure to keep your inner thighs squeezing together. **INHALE** to return to starting position and repeat.

| repeat | 10 times |

BENEFITS OF THE FOOTWORK SERIES

- Strengthens the deep abdominals, especially the transversus abdominis, and the hamstrings.
- Shows how to maintain and stabilize neutral pelvis while moving the legs.

DOS & DON'TS

- Keep your Abdominal Scoop the whole time.

second position
beginning

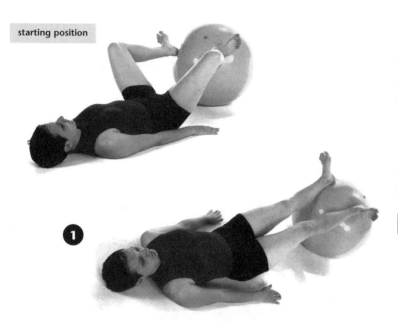

starting position

1

STARTING POSITION: Bend your knees and open your legs hip distance apart. Turn your legs out so that your knees and feet are facing away from each other. **INHALE TO BEGIN.**

1 **EXHALE:** Extend your legs straight out, maintaining the turn-out. **INHALE** to return to starting position and repeat.

repeat	10 times

advanced footwork
advanced

starting position

1

STARTING POSITION: Interlace your fingers behind your head and roll up to the Pilates Abdominal Positioning for a more ab-challenging variation of footwork.

1–2 Repeat First Position, Heels in Parallel and Second Position. You may need to roll down and rest for one or two breaths in between each footwork position.

repeat	10 times

starting position

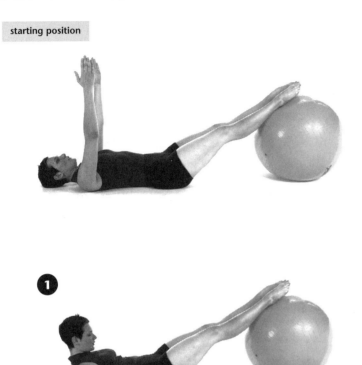

1

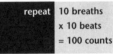

STARTING POSITION: Lie on your back with your arms reaching up to the sky, legs straight and calves resting on the ball. **INHALE TO BEGIN.**

1 **EXHALE:** Roll up to the Pilates Abdominal Positioning, reaching your arms toward the floor. Begin a percussive beating of the arms, small and controlled, a few inches from the floor. Count out 5 beats with your arms and then... **INHALE** through your nose for 5 beats then...**EXHALE** through your mouth, making a shushing sound on every beat for 5 beats...until you count to 100 beats of your arms. Maintain your abdominal positioning the whole time.

repeat	10 breaths
	x 10 beats
	= 100 counts

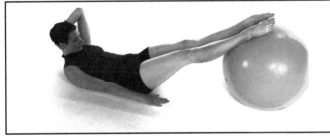

modification

Put one hand behind your head to support your neck if you feel strain.

BENEFITS

- Strengthens the deep neck flexors, abdominals, and hip flexors.
- Stabilizes the lower back.
- Helps you practice percussive breathing.

DOS & DON'TS

- Make sure to keep the Abdominal Scoop.
- Maintain a flat back by scooping the belly in toward the spine; don't let the back arch off the floor.
- Don't let your body roll down from the abdominal positioning; on every exhale make sure your shoulder blades are just off the floor.
- Feel the arms pulsing from the back (latissimus dorsi) rather than from the pectorals.

- Avoid if you have an acute neck injury. This exercise can be hard on the neck, especially if the back of your neck (trapezius muscle) is tight.
- If you have a tight upper back, it may be difficult for you to maintain your upper abdominal curl. Just keep trying!

frog legs

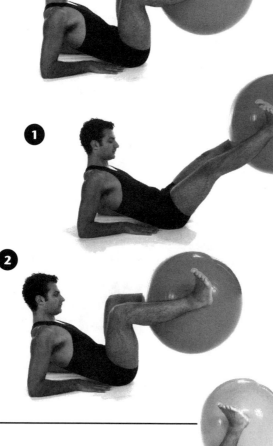

starting position

①

②

STARTING POSITION: Start propped up on your elbows with the ball between your ankles, knees bent into a frog squat, legs slightly turned out. **INHALE TO BEGIN.**

1 EXHALE: Extend your legs diagonally, making sure to pull your belly in. Keep your low back flat on the floor (the lower the legs the more challenging it is to stabilize the core).

2 INHALE: Pull the ball back toward your body.

repeat 6–8 times

advanced variation

Try Frog Legs with your head down on the floor and your Door Frame Arms by your sides. This position is more difficult to stabilize, and therefore more work for your abdominals.

BENEFITS
- Strengthens the abdominals, hip flexors, and inner thighs.
- Stabilizes the low back.

DOS & DON'TS
- Make sure to keep the Abdominal Scoop.
- Maintain a flat low back; don't let the back arch off the floor.

- This exercise requires a lot of core strength. Try it without the ball if you feel strain in your lower back.

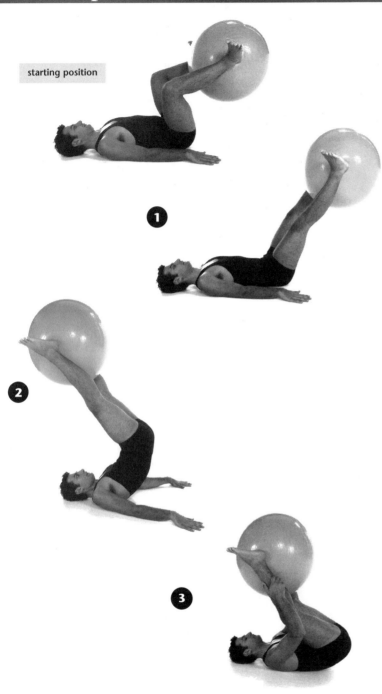

starting position

①

②

③

STARTING POSITION: Lie on your back, arms by your sides, with the ball between your ankles, knees bent into a frog squat, and legs turned out. **INHALE TO BEGIN.**

1 EXHALE: Extend your legs diagonally, making sure to pull your belly in. Keep your low back flat on the floor (the lower the legs the more challenging it is to stabilize the core).

2 INHALE: Lift the ball up and over your head by scooping your belly in and levitating your hips up with your butt muscles. Roll only to the place where you can balance between your shoulder blades.

3 EXHALE: Grab onto your calves as you bend your knees. Pull your belly in as you roll down your spine one vertebra at a time, using the pull of your arms as a counterbalance to increase the stretch in your low back. **INHALE:** Return to frog squat (the starting position).

repeat 3 times

BENEFITS	DOS & DON'TS	IMAGINE
■ Stretches the spine and teaches spinal articulation. ■ Strengthens the core, hip flexors, and inner thighs.	■ Don't roll back so far that you put weight on your neck. ■ Don't do if you have a neck injury.	■ Your butt scooped off the floor from underneath by a hot spatula.

arm reaches

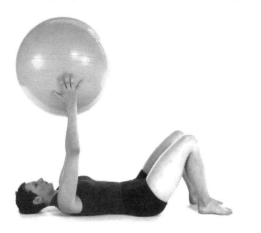

1

STARTING POSITION: Lie on your back with knees bent and feet flat on the floor, hip distance apart.

1 **INHALE:** Reach the ball up to the sky to begin.

2 **EXHALE:** Reach the ball back above your head, knitting your ribcage down to your belly. Only reach back as far as you can maintain the stabilization of your ribs.

repeat **3 times**

2

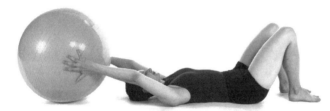

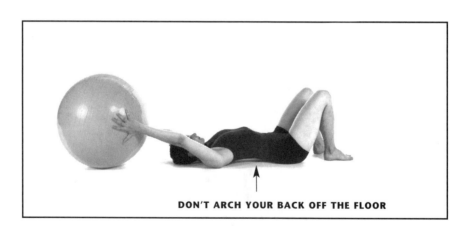

DON'T ARCH YOUR BACK OFF THE FLOOR

BENEFITS	DOS & DON'TS
■ Stabilizes the upper back and ribcage. ■ Stretches the latissimus dorsi and pectoralis minor muscles.	■ Very tight lats or pecs will limit how far you can reach back…but hey, that's why you're doing it! ■ Don't let your upper back arch off the floor as you reach back; instead, engage your upper abdominals to keep the ribcage knitted down.

starting position

STARTING POSITION: Sit up and wrap your legs around the ball in front of you. Try to grab the ball by pulling your heels toward your butt, and hold the ball on either side with your hands.

1 INHALE: Roll back onto your shoulder blades, keeping the ball under the knees.

2 EXHALE: Roll forward as far as you can with control.

repeat 5 times

1

2

variation

Try it without using your hands. "Look, Ma—no hands!"

BENEFITS

- Stretches and articulates the spine.
- Strengthens the abdominals and hamstrings.

DOS & DON'TS

- Don't do if you have a neck injury.
- Even if you don't have a neck injury, don't roll onto your neck; instead, balance between your shoulder blades. See "how to do a rolling exercise" on page 24 for further instructions on how to avoid neck problems.
- If your low back is tight, you will have difficulty rolling smoothly over that area. Slow down and use your Abdominal Scoop to get the low back pressing onto the floor.
- Don't "thump."

IMAGINE

- You are massaging your spine as you roll, trying to get every vertebra in contact with the floor.

roll-up

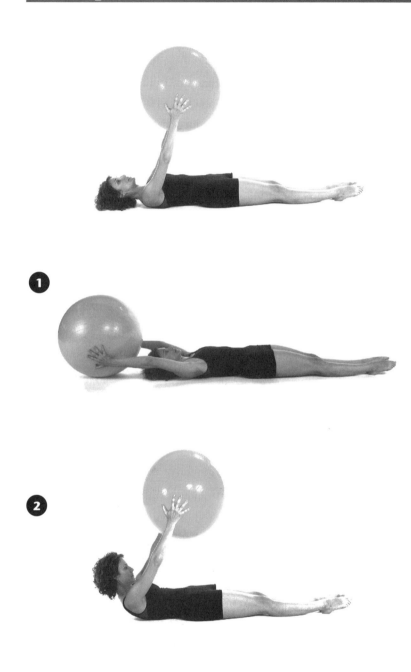

STARTING POSITION: Lie on your back with the ball in your hands reaching up to the sky. Extend your legs straight down on the floor, inner thighs squeezing together in Pilates First Position (slightly turned out). **INHALE TO BEGIN**.

1 As you breathe in, reach the ball back above your head, knit your ribcage down to your belly, and keep your upper back from arching off the floor. Only reach back as far as you can maintain the stabilization in your upper torso.

2 **EXHALE:** Lift the ball up and forward as you roll up, Squeezing a Tangerine under your chin as you sequence the spine off the floor, and squeezing your inner thighs and buns together to assist you in the roll-up.

variations

■ To make the roll-up easier, bend your knees and press your feet into the floor.
■ To make the roll-up more difficult, keep the ball by your ears the whole time.

BENEFITS	DOS & DON'TS	
■ Strengthens abdominals and hip flexors.	■ Don't let your feet come up off the floor; bend your knees if you need to.	but dangerous for your lower back. Make sure you can do this exercise without the ball before attempting it with the extra load.
■ Creates articulation in the spine.	■ Weak abdominals and hip flexors will make this exercise not only difficult	

3 Finish with a C-curve of your whole spine, ball reaching forward. **INHALE:** Hold the stretch.

4 **EXHALE:** Roll down one vertebra at a time, using your Powerhouse to assist you (scooping your belly in and squeezing the inner thighs and butt). Keep the ball reaching forward as a counterbalance.

5 Return to a fully extended position on your back. **INHALE** to begin again.

repeat 4 times

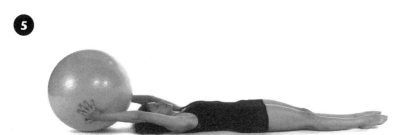

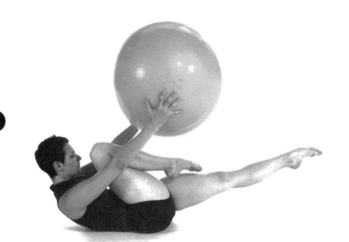

1

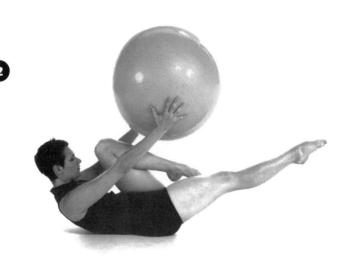

2

STARTING POSITION: Grab the ball and reach it up to the sky as you roll up to the Pilates Abdominal Position. Your shoulder blades are just off the floor.

1 INHALE: Bend your right knee in toward your chest, and extend your left leg long in a diagonal approximately 45 degrees from the floor.

2 EXHALE: Switch legs, keeping your belly pulled in and your low back flat on the floor.

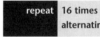

repeat	16 times alternating

BENEFITS	DOS & DON'TS
■ Strengthens neck flexors, abdominals, and hip flexors. ■ Stabilizes the low back.	■ The lower you reach your legs, the harder it is to stabilize the low back, so make sure you keep your low back flat on the floor. Raise the legs up if you cannot maintain a low flat back. ■ Avoid if you have an acute neck injury.

starting position

STARTING POSITION: Lie on your back, knees folded into your chest, and hold the ball in front of your knees. **INHALE TO BEGIN.**

1 **EXHALE:** Keeping your low back flat on the floor and belly scooped in, lengthen both legs diagonally and reach the ball back by your ears.

2 **INHALE**: Return to the starting position.

repeat 5 times

1

2

BENEFITS	DOS & DON'TS	
■ Strengthens neck flexors, abdominals, hip flexors, and lats. ■ Stabilizes the lower back.	■ Don't let your head fall back as you reach your arms by your ears. The only things moving should be your arms and legs! Keep your head perfectly stable by keeping your focus on your belly, not on the moving ball. ■ As in all exercises where your legs are extended to challenge your core,	you must monitor yourself to protect your low back. Only reach your legs as low as you can while still maintaining a flat low back and scooped belly. (See "how to modify to protect your low back" on page 23.) ■ Avoid if you have an acute neck injury.

dead hang fold

starting position

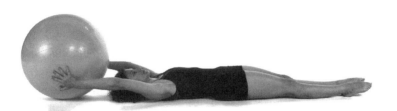

STARTING POSITION: Lie on your back, holding the ball in your hands, arms extended back by your ears and legs straight in front of you in Pilates First Position. **INHALE TO BEGIN.**

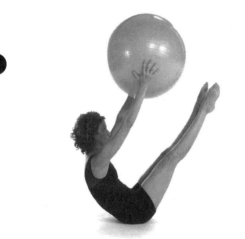

1 EXHALE: Scoop your belly in and squeeze your butt to initiate folding your body in half, bringing your arms and legs up to the sky.

2 INHALE: Unfold your body, keeping your arms by your ears as you lower your legs and upper body down toward the floor. Come down almost to a "dead hang."

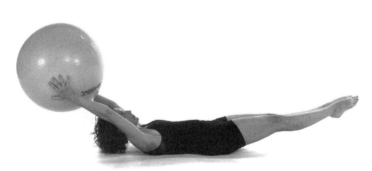

BENEFITS	DOS & DON'TS
■ Strengthens neck flexors, abdominals, hip flexors, and lats.	■ Only lower your legs as far as you can maintain a flat lower back; no arching off the mat! ■ Don't use the ball if you feel strain in your low back. This is an intense core challenge!

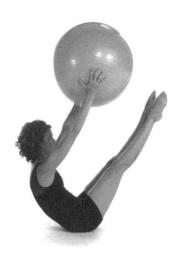

3 **EXHALE:** Fold in half again. Repeat this part of the exercise two more times.

4 At the top of your final repetition, switch the ball from your hands to between your ankles.

5 **INHALE:** Unfold your body, keeping your arms by your ears as you lower your legs and upper body down toward the floor. Come down almost to a "dead hang." Repeat this part of the exercise three times.

repeat	3 times then switch ball to feet

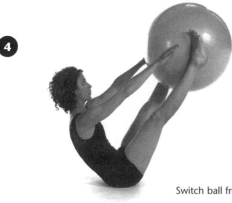

Switch ball from hands to feet.

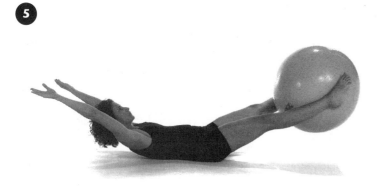

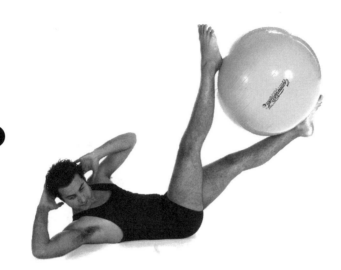

1

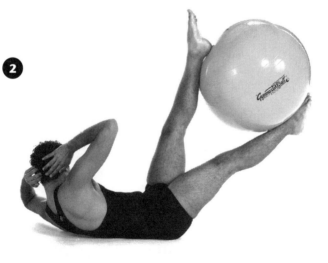

2

STARTING POSITION: Lie on your back with the ball between your ankles and legs reaching up toward the sky. Interlace your fingers behind your head and roll up to the Pilates Abdominal Positioning. **INHALE TO BEGIN.**

1 **EXHALE**: Reach one elbow toward the opposite knee as you rotate the ball between your legs.

2 **INHALE:** Alternate sides.

repeat	16 times alternating

BENEFITS

- Strengthens neck flexors, inner thighs, hip flexors, and abdominals (especially the internal and external obliques).

DOS & DON'TS

- Don't allow your upper body to roll down from the Pilates Abdominal Positioning. Keep the shoulder blades off the floor the whole time.
- Keep your elbows wide so that you are twisting your torso, not your arms. You don't need to actually touch the opposite knee.
- Think of rotating your trunk from the back, imagining your shoulder blades wrapping around to the front as you twist the upper body.
- Upper back tightness will limit your ability to maintain your curl up.
- Avoid if you have an acute neck injury.

IMAGINE

- You are rotating around a stake that anchors your sternum to the floor.

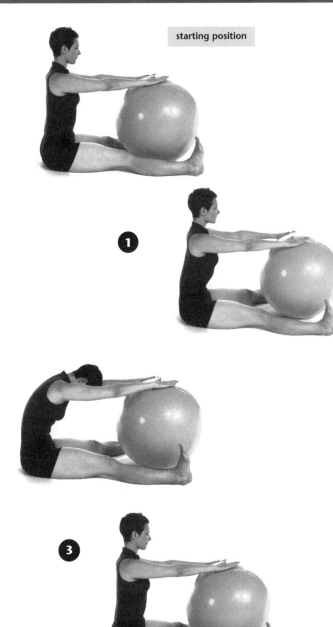

starting position

STARTING POSITION: Sit up with your legs extended and the ball between them. Extend your Door Frame Arms on top of the ball, shoulder distance apart, palms down. Lift your belly off your legs, and engage your glutes by pulling your sits bones together. **INHALE TO BEGIN.**

1–2 **EXHALE**: Pull your navel in toward your spine as you round your back up and forward into a C-curve, starting from the base of your spine and sequencing up to your head. Your back should end in the shape of a capital "C."

3 **INHALE:** Stack up from the base of your spine, letting your head be the last thing to rise. Sit up tall to start again. **EXHALE**, let the shoulders drop back down, and repeat.

repeat 3 times

BENEFITS	DOS & DON'TS	IMAGINE
■ Stretches the whole spine from coccyx to occiput. ■ Creates length in spine while rounding forward. ■ Allows you to practice the C-curve. ■ Articulates and stacks the spine.	■ Tight hamstrings will limit your ability to sit up straight with your legs straight in front of you. Bend your knees to ease the hamstrings.	■ You must lift up and over a barrel that sits on your lap in order to reach forward.

starting position

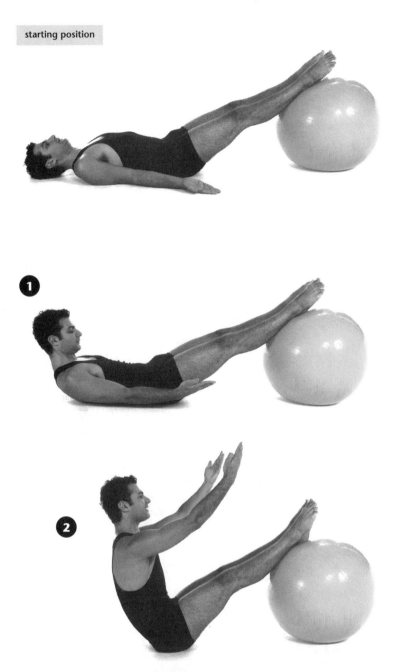

①

②

STARTING POSITION: Lie on your back with your legs on the ball in Pilates First Position (turned out and inner thighs squeezing together), arms by your sides, palms facing up. Your calves should be making contact with ball. **INHALE TO BEGIN.**

1 **EXHALE:** Squeeze a Tangerine under your chin as you lift your head off the floor, pulling your shoulder blades down as you reach forward with your arms. Scoop your belly in and squeeze your butt and inner thighs together as you roll all the way up to your balance point, stopping just before you reach your tailbone.

2 At the top of the Teaser, your arms reach up and forward as you try to lift your chest while keeping your low belly scooped in. **INHALE** at the top.

BENEFITS	DOS & DON'TS	IMAGINE
■ Strengthens abdominals and hip flexors. ■ Articulates the spine.	■ Tight hamstrings will make this exercise much more difficult; if you suffer from this, try the variation. ■ Make sure to keep the shoulders down away from the ears.	■ An energy force pulls the shoulder blades down the back as you initiate the roll up into your Teaser, then travels down and around to the front as you scoop your belly in. Back to front.

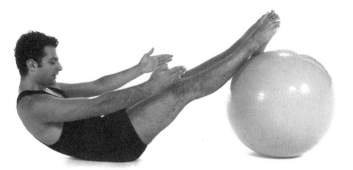

3 EXHALE: Scoop your belly in and squeeze your butt and inner thighs together as you roll all the way down your spine, allowing your arms to trail down to the starting position. **INHALE** and repeat.

repeat 4 times

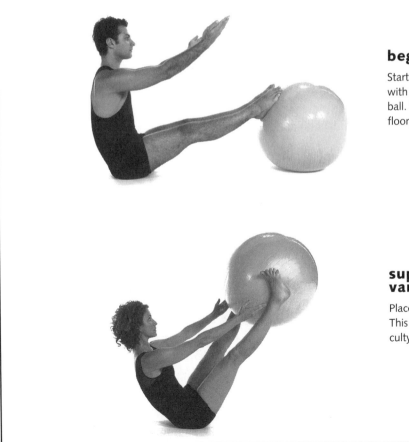

beginner variation

Start with the ball farther away, with the soles of your feet on the ball. The lower your legs are to the floor, the easier the Teaser will be.

super-advanced variation

Place the ball between your legs. This exponentially increases the difficulty of this exercise!

rollover

starting position

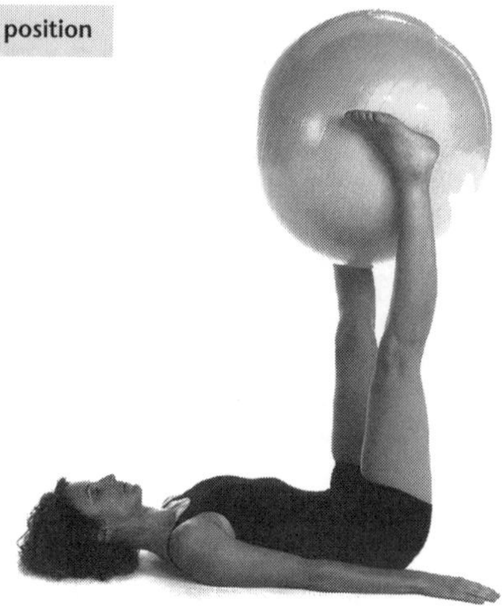

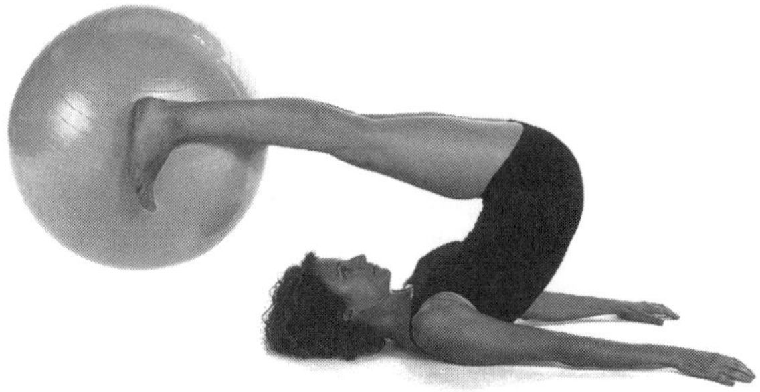

STARTING POSITION: Lie on your back with legs straight up toward the sky, ball between your ankles and Door Frame Arms down by your sides, palms facing down. **INHALE TO BEGIN.**

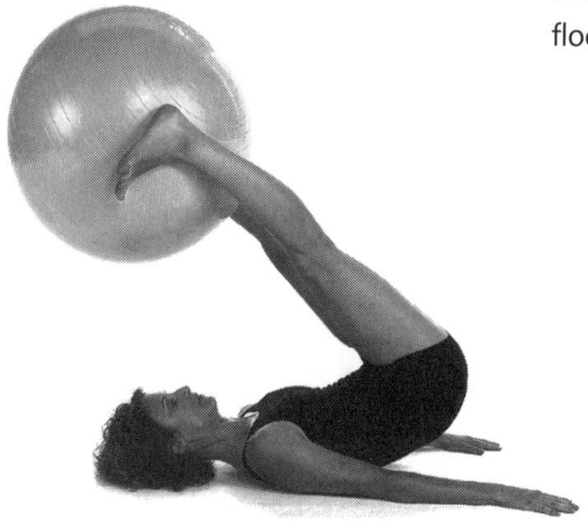

1 Scoop your belly in as you lift the ball up and over your head.

2 Reach the ball to the wall behind you, with your weight balanced between your shoulder blades. Press your arms down onto the floor to help control the movement.

1

2

BENEFITS	DOS & DON'TS	
■ Stretches and articulates the spine. ■ Strengthens the abdominals, inner thighs, triceps, and lats.	■ Press the arms down to control your movements, but don't let the shoulders hunch up by your ears—keep them stabilized down the back. ■ Don't roll onto your neck.	■ Try to articulate through each vertebra by pulling your belly in and pressing the low back onto the floor as you roll back.

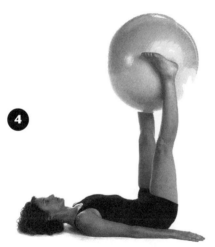

3 **EXHALE:** Flex your feet, reaching your heels long toward the back wall as you roll down your spine, one vertebra at a time.

4 Control the movement with your Abdominal Scoop until your hips reach down to the floor. **INHALE** and repeat.

repeat	4 times

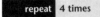

super-advanced variation

To increase the abdominal challenge, let the ball drop forward before rolling over again. But only go as far as you can maintain a flat low back on the floor.

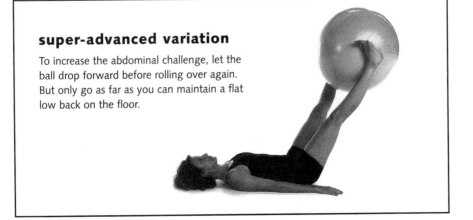

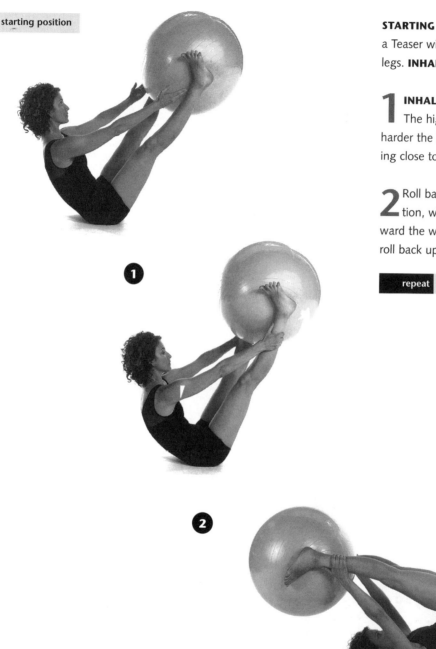

starting position

1

2

STARTING POSITION: Roll up into a Teaser with the ball between your legs. **INHALE TO BEGIN.**

1 **INHALE:** Grab onto your legs. The higher you grab, the harder the balance. Begin by holding close to your knees.

2 Roll back to your Rollover position, with the ball reaching toward the wall behind you. **EXHALE,** roll back up, and repeat.

repeat | 5 times

BENEFITS

- Stretches and articulates the spine.
- Strengthens the abdominals, triceps, and lats.

DOS & DON'TS

- Go slowly so that you can feel the articulation of the spine.
- Don't roll onto your neck; instead, balance between your shoulder blades.

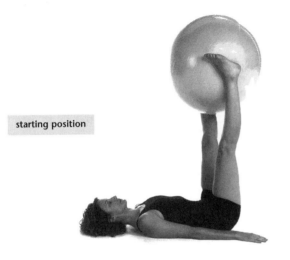

starting position

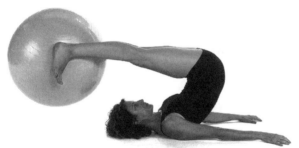

①

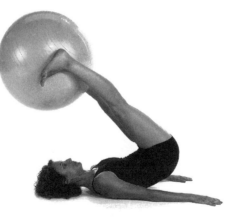

②

STARTING POSITION: Lie on your back with the ball between your legs and Door Frame Arms on the floor beside you.

1 INHALE: Scoop your belly in as you lift the ball up and over your head. Reach the ball to the wall behind you, with your weight balanced between your shoulder blades. Press your arms down onto the floor to help control the movement.

2 EXHALE: Flex your feet, reaching your heels long toward the back wall as you roll down your spine, one vertebra at a time. Control the movement with your Abdominal Scoop until your hips reach down to the floor.

variation

This is a great way to combine three advanced exercises. If you do this sequence, there's no need to do the exercises separately.

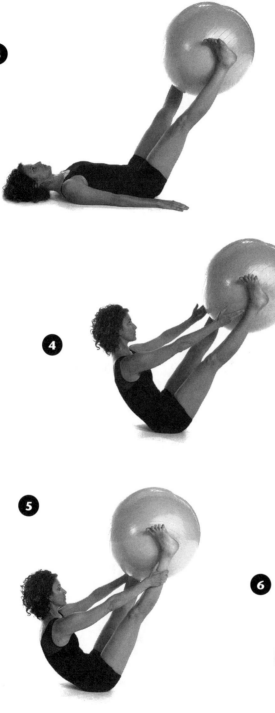

3 Allow your legs to slowly drop a few degrees toward the floor, keeping your low back flat on the floor. **INHALE.**

4 **EXHALE:** Roll up into the Teaser: Squeeze a Tangerine under your chin as you lift your head off the floor, pulling your shoulder blades down as you reach forward with your arms. Scoop your belly in and squeeze your butt and inner thighs together as you roll all the way up to your balance point, stopping just before you reach your tailbone. At the top of the Teaser, your arms reach up and forward as you try to lift your chest while keeping your low belly scooped in. **INHALE** at the top.

5 Grab onto your legs.

6 **INHALE:** Roll back to your Rollover position, with the ball reaching toward the wall behind you.

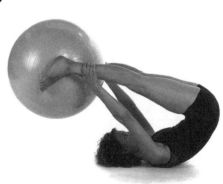

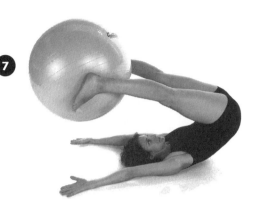

7 **EXHALE:** Release your arms down onto the floor above your head.

8 Roll down one vertebra at a time until your hips reach the floor.

9 **INHALE:** Allow your legs to drop a few degrees and roll back up into your Teaser.

10 **INHALE:** Grab onto your legs. Repeat steps 6–9 three times. Do the Open Leg Rocker three times.

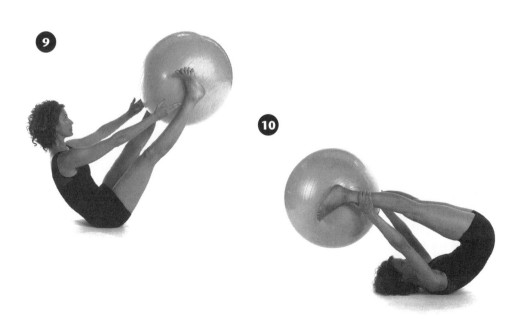

around the world

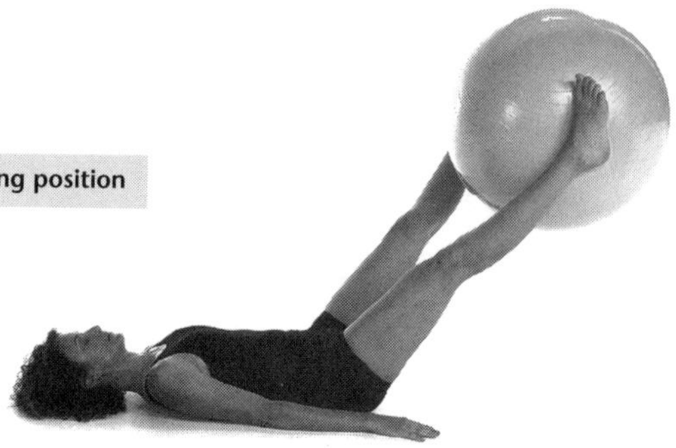

starting position

STARTING POSITION: Lie on your back with your legs up in a diagonal, the ball between your legs and Door Frame Arms down by your side, palms facing down. Make sure to keep your belly pulled in and your back flat on the floor. **INHALE TO BEGIN.**

1–2 **EXHALE:** Begin a large circle with the ball, lifting your hips to the left.

❶

❷

BENEFITS	DOS & DON'TS
■ Stretches and articulates the spine. ■ Strengthens the abdominals, especially the obliques.	■ Don't roll onto your neck. ■ Keep pulling navel to spine. ■ Press Door Frame Arms onto the floor to help stabilize you.

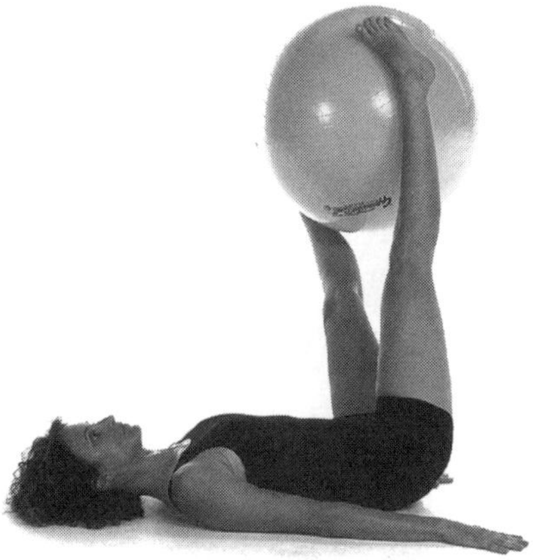

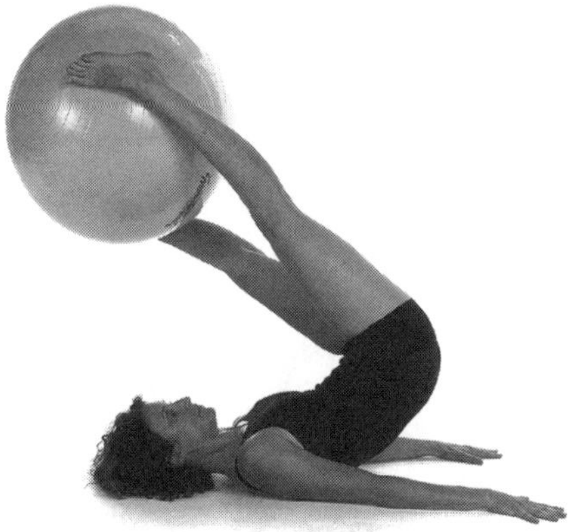

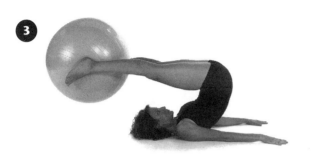

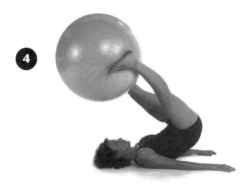

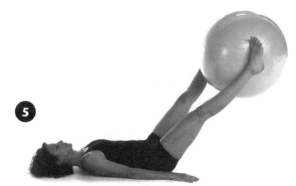

3 Continue the circle, lifting the ball up and over your head.

4 Continue the circle, now coming down toward your right.

5 Finish the circle in the starting position. **INHALE** and reverse directions.

repeat | 4 times

starting position

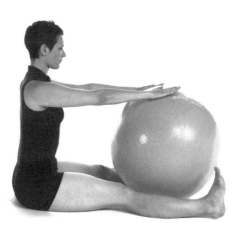

STARTING POSITION: Sit up tall with the ball between your legs, squeezing your inner thighs together, Door Frame Arms on top of the ball. Lengthen your spine by lifting your belly up off your hips. **INHALE TO BEGIN.**

1 EXHALE: Thread your left arm under the right. Twist from your middle, reaching your left arm to the right foot.

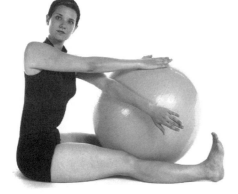

2 Put some pressure on the ball to help increase the stretch, and think of sawing off your pinkie toe with your pinkie finger in two gentle movements. Reach the right arm back behind you. Keep both hips grounded on the floor.

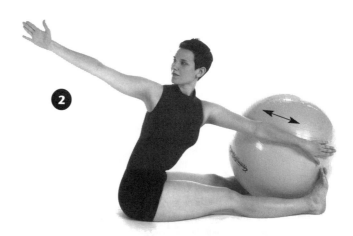

BENEFITS	DOS & DON'TS	IMAGINE
■ Stretches the back muscles, especially the quadratus lumborum. ■ Increases rotation in the spine.	■ Make sure both hips stay grounded for optimal stretch. ■ Keep the ball secure by squeezing it between your inner thighs.	■ Your spine is a DNA spiral.

4 **INHALE:** Thread the right arm through to other side of the ball.

5 **EXHALE:** Perform the movement on the other side. **INHALE** and repeat.

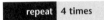

repeat | 4 times

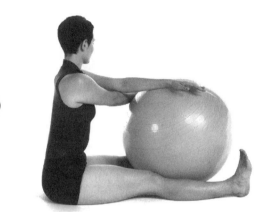

4

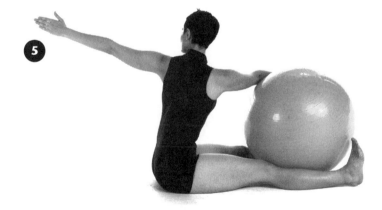

5

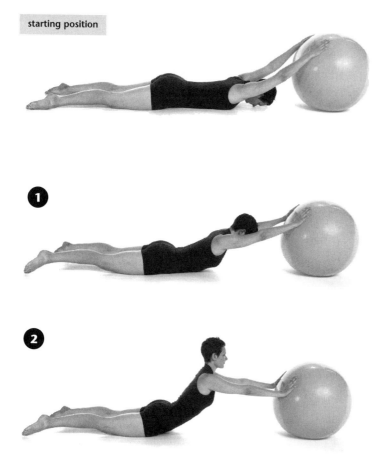

starting position

STARTING POSITION: Lie on your belly with your face on the floor, arms up on the ball a little wider than shoulder distance apart, legs turned out and hip distance apart. **INHALE TO BEGIN.**

1 EXHALE: Pull the shoulders down away from your ears, which will move the ball slightly toward you, then raise your head and upper body up off the floor.

2 INHALE: Come all the way up, pressing your arms down into the ball. Make sure to protect your lower back by scooping your belly up off the floor, pressing your pubic bone down on the floor, and squeezing your butt. **EXHALE** and return to the floor. **INHALE** to begin again.

repeat **4 times**

variation

To lessen the intensity of the shoulder stretch and to decrease the compression in your low back, lower your hands to the sides of the ball.

BENEFITS	DOS & DON'TS	IMAGINE
■ Strengthens back and neck extensors. ■ Stretches lats and pecs.	■ Make sure to keep the shoulders down and the neck long. ■ If you feel compression in your lower back, scoop your belly in as much as you can. If you still feel compression, don't come up so high. ■ Don't let your head be a Broken Bud at the top of your spine. The head should always follow the arc of the spine. (See page 19 for further instructions.)	■ As you lift your head you are watching an ant crawling away from you on the floor. (This image will keep your head and neck on the right track.)

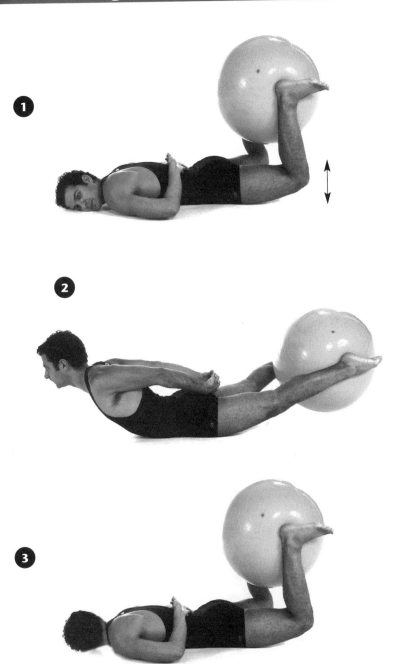

STARTING POSITION: Lie with your head to one side, your knees bent 90 degrees and the ball between your ankles. Your fingers should be interlaced behind you, with your elbows bent as much as possible and relaxed by your sides.

1 INHALE TO BEGIN. Squeeze your ankles together as you pulse the ball up to the sky three times.

2 EXHALE: Keep the thighs lifted up off the floor as you extend your legs behind you, straightening your arms back to lift your head and upper body off the floor, stretching your chest open.

3 INHALE: Return to the floor, with your head facing the opposite way, knees bent and arms bending back to the starting position. **EXHALE** and repeat.

repeat	4 times

BENEFITS

- Strengthens the butt, hamstrings, back, and neck extensors.
- Stretches the chest and belly.

DOS & DON'TS

- To avoid low back compression and maximize butt work, don't let your back arch when doing the pulses; instead, keep your pelvis tucked under, pressing your pubic bone down and lifting your belly up off the floor.

hinge curl roll-down

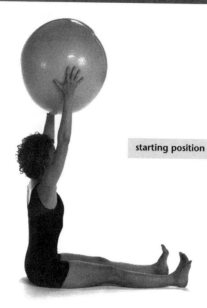

starting position

STARTING POSITION: Sit up with your legs straight in front of you, hip distance apart, feet flexed. With the ball between your hands, reach your arms up to the sky.

1 INHALE: Lift up through your hips and scoop the belly as you hinge back as far as you can, keeping your spine straight.

2 EXHALE: Scoop your belly in. Shovel your pelvis under, creating a C-curve in your low back, and roll down one vertebra at a time, reaching your ball up and slightly forward of your body.

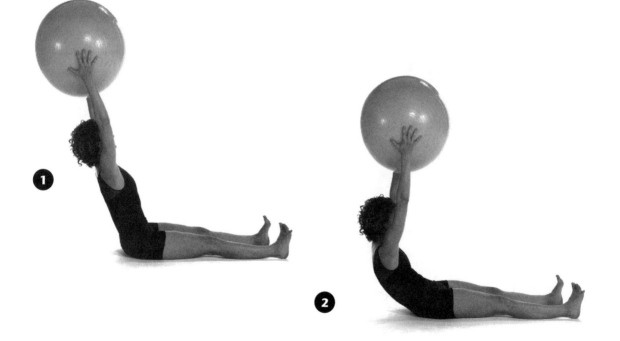

BENEFITS	DOS & DON'TS
■ Strengthens abdominals and hip flexors. ■ Articulates the spine.	■ Activate your legs on the roll down and the roll up by reaching long through your heels. ■ Remember: this is the hardest roll-up!

hinge curl roll-down

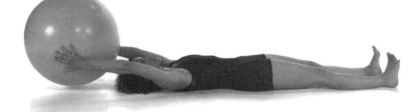

3

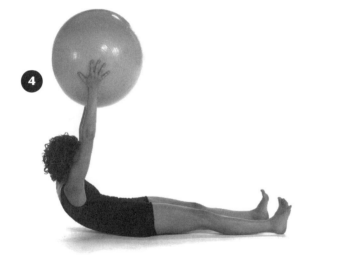

4

3 INHALE: Finish flat on your back with arms and ball reaching back behind you.

4 EXHALE: Lift the ball up to the sky. Squeeze a Tangerine under your chin to lift your head and begin to roll up, reaching the ball up and forward.

5 INHALE: Stack your spine, reaching the ball up to the sky. **EXHALE** and repeat.

repeat	4 times

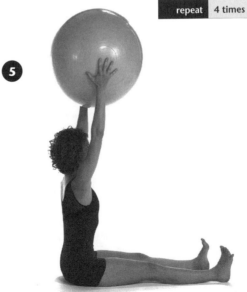

5

variation

- Some people find it easier to roll up with knees bent.

STARTING POSITION: Lie on your back, with your legs straight and resting together up on the ball, arms by your sides, palms facing down. **INHALE TO BEGIN.**

1 **EXHALE:** Scooping your belly in, coccyx curl one vertebra up at a time until your hips are up in a straight line with your legs.

2 **INHALE:** Hold the bridge. **EXHALE** and roll back down to the floor, articulating one vertebra at a time. **INHALE** and repeat.

repeat | 4 times

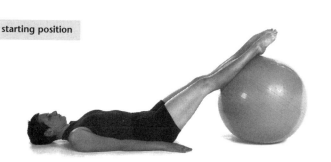

starting position

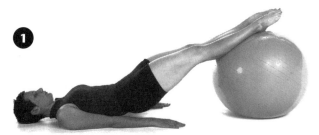

1

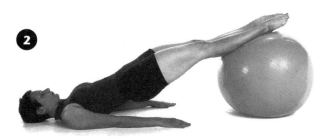

2

BENEFITS OF THE BRIDGE SERIES	DOS & DON'TS
■ Strengthens hamstrings and butt. ■ Articulates and stabilizes spine. ■ One-legged bridges challenge stability and strengthen the gluteus medius.	■ Don't roll up so high that your back arches; keep your hips in line with your body, making a straight line from your shoulders to your toes. ■ The farther the ball is away from you the harder it is to stabilize, so place the ball accordingly.

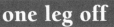
starting position

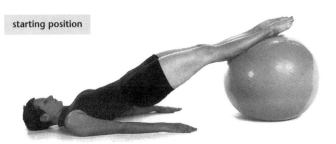

STARTING POSITION: Begin in the regular two-legged bridge. **INHALE TO BEGIN.**

1 **EXHALE:** Bend your right knee and lift it up to the sky.

2 **INHALE:** Hold. As you exhale, think of giving an extra hip lift, as if you are reaching your toes to the heavens. Place your leg back on the ball and alternate sides. **INHALE** and repeat.

repeat	4 times alternating

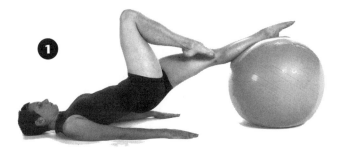
1

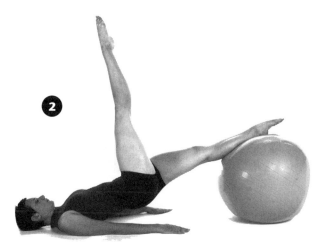
2

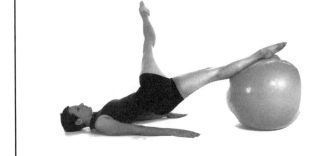

variation

To increase the challenge you can add a hip twist, come back to center, and replace the leg back on the ball. Then switch sides. Repeat 2 times.

bridge series

bent-knee bridge

intermediate

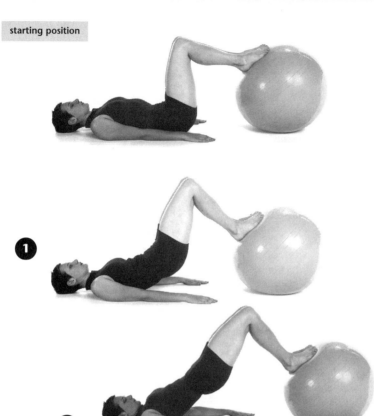

starting position

This variation is quite a workout for your hamstrings as well as a great stabilization exercise for the knee.

STARTING POSITION: Place your feet on the ball, knees bent at an acute angle. **INHALE TO BEGIN.**

1 **EXHALE:** Scoop your belly in toward your spine. Roll up one vertebra at a time, keeping the ball stable underneath you.

2 **INHALE** at the top of your Bridge and hold for one full breath.
EXHALE to retrograde the movement down to the floor.
INHALE and repeat.

repeat 4 times

hamstring stretch

beginning

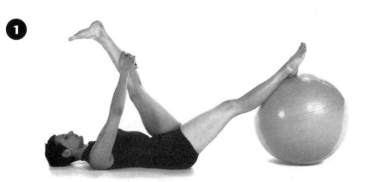

After doing many Bridges, you may need this hamstring stretch.

1 Lift one leg off the ball and hold it with your hands above the knee. Try to keep the leg straight by engaging the quad muscles in the front of the leg. Breathe deeply and on every exhale try to increase the stretch by pulling the leg closer to your body. Make sure to keep your shoulders down the back, elbows wide, using your biceps to pull the leg.

repeat 4 times

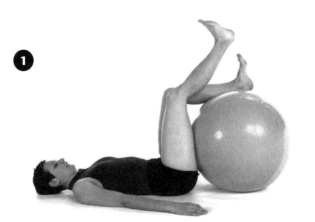

STARTING POSITION: Lie on your back with your knees bent and calves on the ball, feet flexed. **INHALE TO BEGIN**.

1–2 **EXHALE:** Start drumming the ball with your heels slowly at first, then try to drum as fast as possible, making very small movements.

repeat 30–50 times

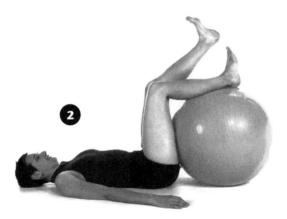

BENEFITS	DOS & DON'TS	IMAGINE
■ Strengthens the hamstrings. ■ Releases pent-up rage.	■ Keep pulling the ball in toward your thighs if it starts rolling away. ■ Maintain Neutral Spine and scooped-in belly.	■ You are hammering away with your heels, trying to pop the ball

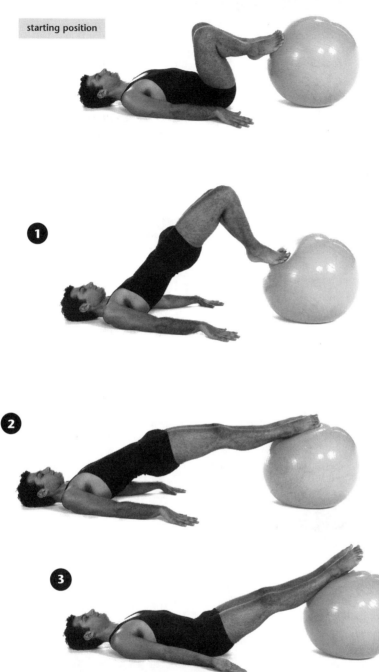

starting position

1

2

3

STARTING POSITION: Lie on your back, Door Frame Arms by your sides, legs in a frog squat, knees bent all the way and turned out a little wider than your hips. The balls of your feet are up on the ball, and your heels are off the ball, squeezing together. **INHALE TO BEGIN**.

1 EXHALE: Scoop your belly in and coccyx curl your hips up until they are all the way in line with your thighs. Your whole torso should be making a straight line from your shoulders to your hips. Keep your heels up off the ball and squeezing together. Your knees should be open a little wider than your hips. Hold this position for one full breath.

2 INHALE: Straighten your legs, keeping your hips up in the Bridge.

3 EXHALE: Roll down on vertebra at a time until your back is flat on the floor. **INHALE.**

BENEFITS	DOS & DON'TS	IMAGINE
■ Strengthens hamstrings, glutes, and inner thighs. ■ Stretches hip flexors and quads. ■ Teaches articulation of spine.	■ When you are up in the Bridge, knit the ribcage down. ■ Take any arch out of your back, scoop your belly in, and squeeze your butt. ■ Think of pressing your hips up from your butt.	■ **George Foreman Grill**: You are being flattened from the front and back of your body, like a *croque monsieur* inside a George Foreman Grill.

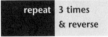

4 **EXHALE:** Coccyx curl back up to your bridge, keeping legs straight.

5 **INHALE:** Keeping your hips lifted, bend your knees back into the frog squat, pulling the ball toward you, keeping your heels off the ball, squeezing them together.

6 **EXHALE:** Roll down on vertebra at a time, coming back to the starting position.

repeat	3 times & reverse

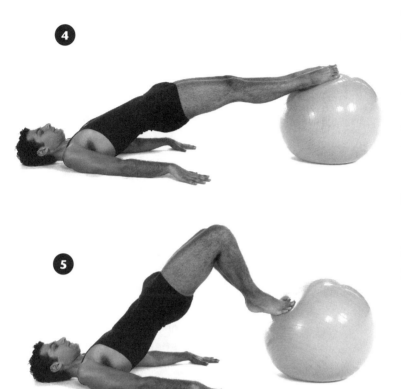

4

5

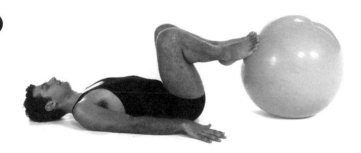

6

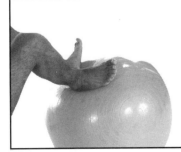

modification

Snake: This is an easier version of the Semi-Circle because you don't have to keep your heels up off the ball. Instead, perform the same exercise but keep your heels down on the ball in Pilates First Position.

control back

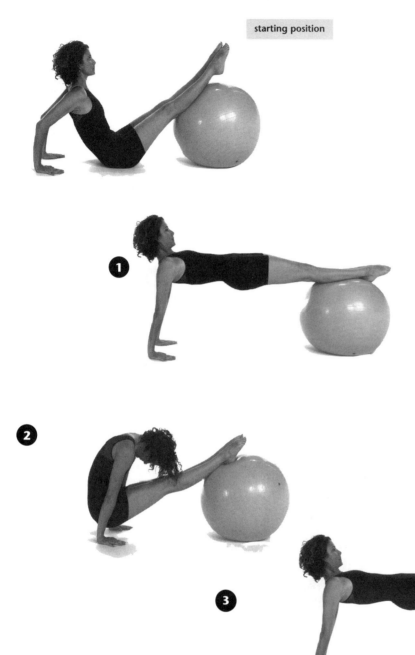

starting position

STARTING POSITION: Sit propped up on your arms with hands on either side of your hips, fingers spread and facing forward, and the ball under your calves.

1 INHALE: Keep the legs and arms straight as you lift your hips up so that your whole body is like a table top.

2 EXHALE: Scoop your belly in as you pull the ball toward you, allowing your body to fold in half.

3 INHALE: Come back to the table top position, squeezing your butt to elevate the hips. **EXHALE** and repeat.

repeat | 4 times

BENEFITS

- Strengthens the arms, legs, back, butt, and belly.
- Teaches balance and control.

DOS & DON'TS

- Keep your fingers spread and pressed into the floor to lessen wrist compression.

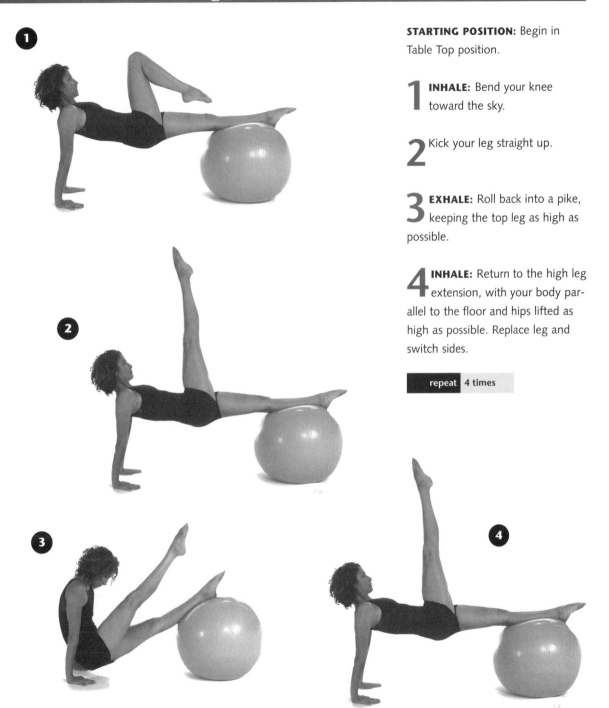

STARTING POSITION: Begin in Table Top position.

1 **INHALE:** Bend your knee toward the sky.

2 Kick your leg straight up.

3 **EXHALE:** Roll back into a pike, keeping the top leg as high as possible.

4 **INHALE:** Return to the high leg extension, with your body parallel to the floor and hips lifted as high as possible. Replace leg and switch sides.

| repeat | 4 times |

BENEFITS

- Strengthens the arms, legs, back, butt, and belly.
- Teaches balance and control.

DOS & DON'TS

- Keep your fingers spread and pressing into the floor to lessen wrist compression.

side kicks

starting position

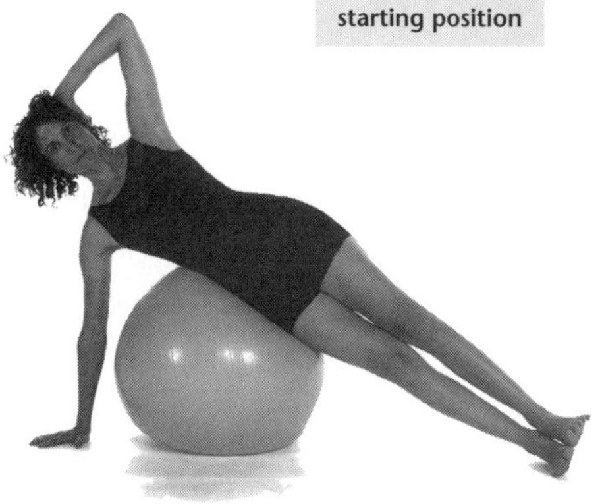

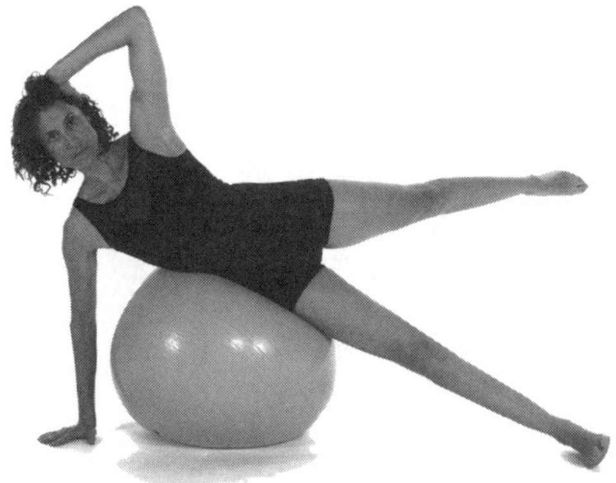

STARTING POSITION: Lie sideways with one hip supported on the ball and your body and limbs in the shape of a star, with the same side arm and leg making contact with the floor to stabilize.

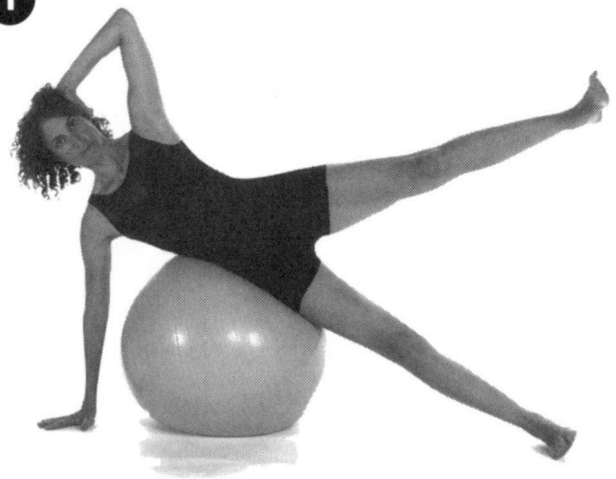

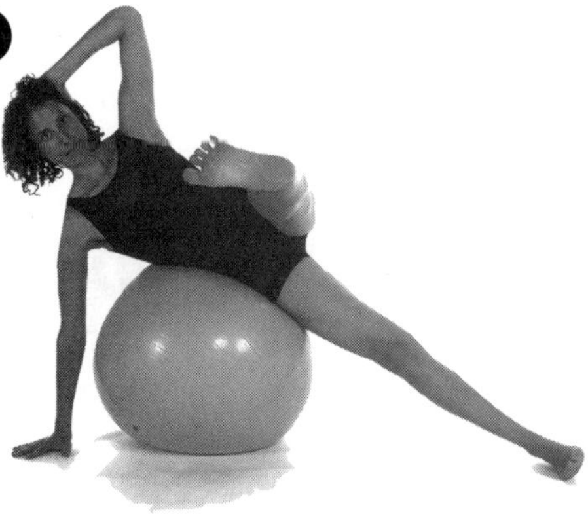

1 Raise the top leg to the sky.

2 **INHALE:** Flex the foot that's up in the air as you kick it forward, making a double pulse at the end of the movement.

3 **EXHALE:** Point the foot as you kick it back, again making a double pulse at the end of the movement. **INHALE** and kick forward to repeat.

repeat | 10 times

BENEFITS	DOS & DON'TS
■ Strengthens the butt and belly.	■ Keep your body stable.
■ Teaches balance and control.	■ Don't kick so far behind you that your back arches.

starting position

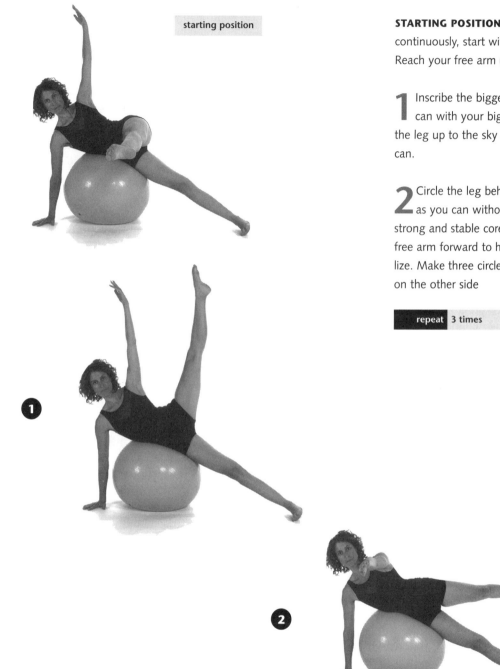

STARTING POSITION: Breathing continuously, start with a side kick. Reach your free arm up to the sky.

1 Inscribe the biggest circle you can with your big toe, reaching the leg up to the sky as far as you can.

2 Circle the leg behind you as far as you can without losing your strong and stable core. Reach your free arm forward to help you stabilize. Make three circles, then repeat on the other side

repeat 3 times

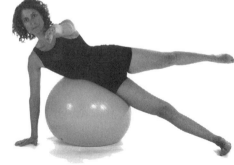

BENEFITS	DOS & DON'TS
■ Strengthens the butt and belly.	■ Keep your body stable.
■ Teaches balance and control.	■ Don't kick so far behind you that your back arches.

①

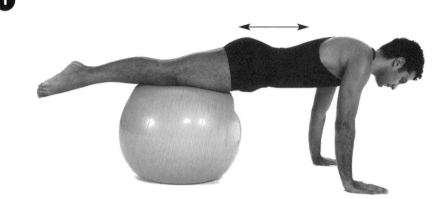

STARTING POSITION: Lie prone on the ball with your hands on the floor in front of you and the ball under your knees. Slowly walk forward on your hands as you come into the Plank position. Your whole body from shoulders to toes should make a level plane. Legs should be straight and pulled together from the inner thigh, arms straight and strong, and hands facing forward with fingers spread.

1 Breathing continuously, slowly roll forward and back on your arms five times, making micro movements, allowing no change in your Plank. Keep your belly scooped in and your buttocks toned. Only move six inches—at the most—forward and back.

| repeat | 5 times |

BENEFITS OF THE PLANK SERIES	DOS & DON'TS	IMAGINE
■ Strengthens the arms, back, and core. ■ Teaches balance and control.	■ Don't allow your Plank to sag. Instead, pull your belly up and in and squeeze your butt. ■ If you feel discomfort in your low back, then don't roll out so far away from the ball—keep it closer to you until you develop the necessary core strength. ■ Don't let your head drop as you go down in your push-up.	■ You are a plank of wood and someone is going to step on your low back area. Make sure to feel the support so your plank doesn't break!

STARTING POSITION: Start in the Plank.

1 Breathe slowly and continuously as you do a set of push-ups. Allow your elbows to bend sideways as you go down in the push-up. The farther away you are from the ball, the greater the stability challenge.

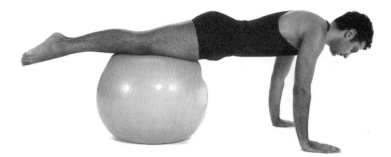

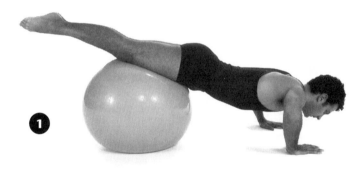

repeat 8–10 times

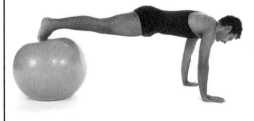

advanced variation

■ For a huge stability challenge, place your toes on the ball and do your push ups.

STARTING POSITION: The Plank with the knees on top of the ball. **INHALE TO BEGIN.**

1 **EXHALE:** Pull the ball toward you with straight legs.

2 Scoop your belly in and fold your body like a pike. Make sure to keep your legs perfectly straight. **INHALE** and return to the Plank.

repeat 6–8 times

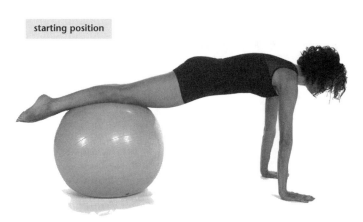

starting position

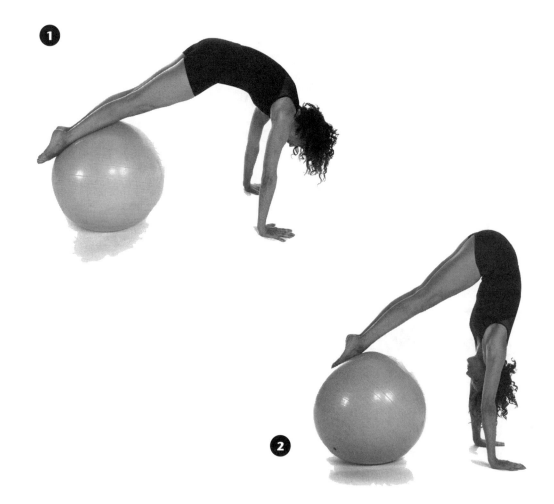

1

2

starting position

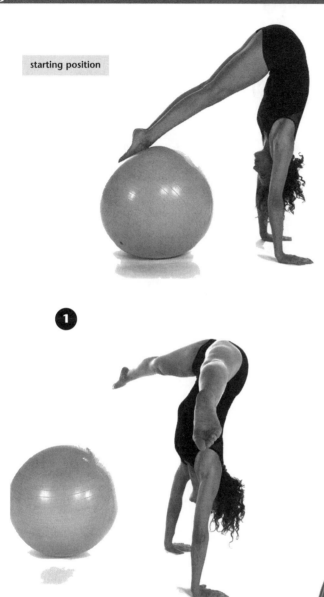

Once you have mastered the Jackknife and can hold the pike position with your hips on top of your shoulders, then you are ready to try going up into a handstand.

STARTING POSITION: From Jackknife keep rolling forward ever so slowly until you are able to lift the legs off the ball.

1 As your legs come off the ball, allow them to open wide, making a circle that finishes at the top with the legs squeezing together and pointing straight up to the sky.

2 See if you can hold your handstand while continuing to breathe. Be careful as you come out of your handstand—don't land back on the ball! Come out of the handstand by kicking one leg down at a time, and come to a standing position. No need to repeat!

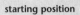
starting position

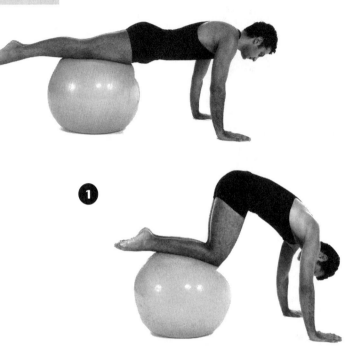

1

2

STARTING POSITION: The Plank with your knees on top of the ball. **INHALE TO BEGIN.**

1 EXHALE: Pull the ball forward with your knees by scooping your belly in and folding in the middle, allowing your knees to bend.

2 Finish in a fetal position on top of the ball. **INHALE** and return to the Plank.

repeat **8 times**

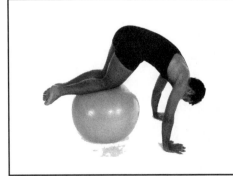

oblique variation

Instead of pulling the ball forward in a straight line, allow your knees to direct the ball slightly off center as you pull it in toward you, stopping at the fetal position. Then return to the Plank by sending the ball out the opposite direction, making an oval pathway with the ball. Make sure you keep your hips above the ball at all times. If you let the hips drop down, you may find yourself on the floor!

one leg off (control front)   *advanced*

starting position

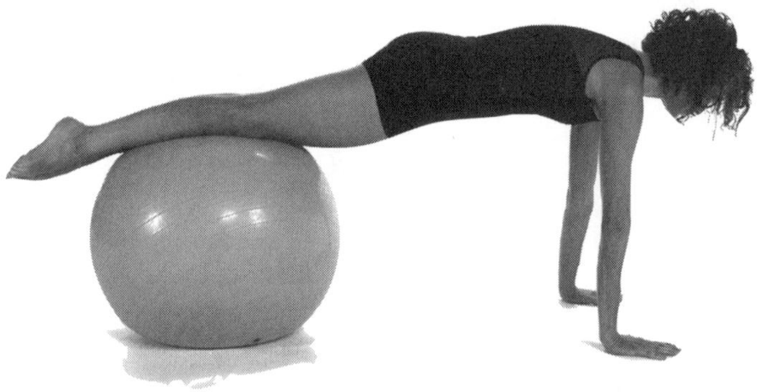

STARTING POSITION: Begin in the Plank, breathing continuously.

1 Lift up one leg and roll forward, pointing your toes.

2 As you roll back, flex your feet. Repeat three times back and forth, pointing as you roll forward, flexing as you roll back, then replace the leg on the ball and switch sides.

repeat	3 times each leg

1

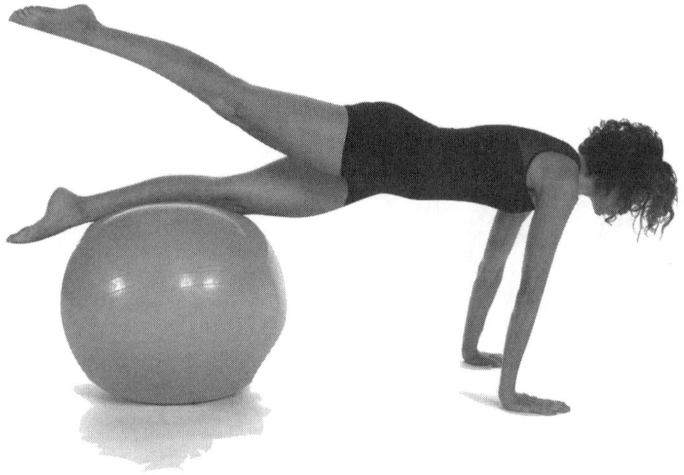

2

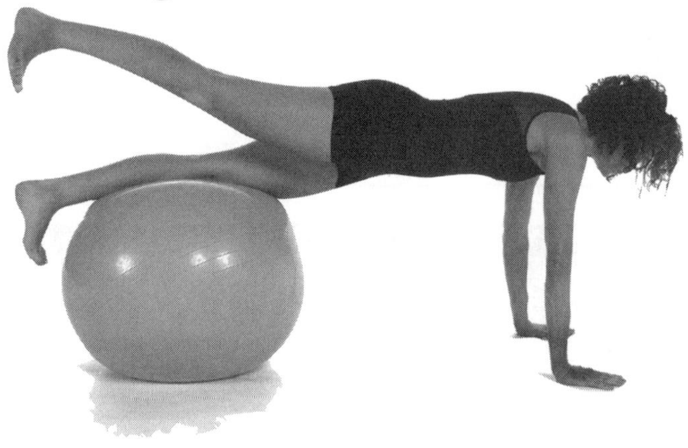

starting position

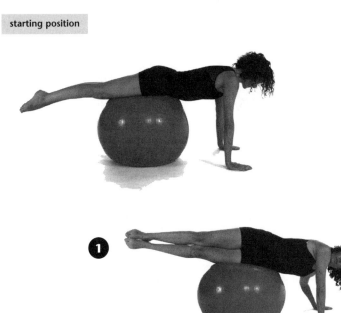

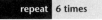

STARTING POSITION: The Plank position with hips on top of the ball, hands on the floor in front of you, fingers spread, arms strong and straight. **INHALE TO BEGIN.**

1 EXHALE: Twist your hips 90 degrees so that your hips are turned at a right angle to your shoulders. Keep your legs straight, strong, and pulled together.

2 INHALE: Return to start position. **EXHALE** and roll to the other side.

repeat 6 times

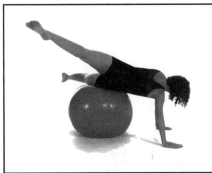

variation

Hip Twist with Split: Try splitting your legs open when you twist, reaching your bottom leg forward and your top leg back. This adds an even greater stretch for your spine.

BENEFITS	DOS & DON'TS
■ Strengthens arms, back, and core. ■ Stretches the spine.	■ Make the movement percussive and controlled, stopping when you've hit the flat place on the side of your hip. If you go too slow you may keep rolling....

starting position

1

2

STARTING POSITION: The Plank position with hips on top of the ball, hands on the floor in front of you, fingers spread, arms strong and straight. **INHALE** into a high Swan, extending your spine and lifting your upper back and head.

1 **EXHALE:** Bend your elbows so that your upper body comes closer to the floor. Keep your elbows glued to the sides of your ribcage and keep your chest open. Lift your legs up toward the sky behind you, keeping the inner thighs squeezing together.

2 **INHALE:** Straighten your arms, coming up into a high Swan, lifting and opening your chest, leading up with your head. **INHALE** and repeat.

repeat **8 times**

BENEFITS	DOS & DON'TS
■ Opens the chest and reverses hunchback posture. ■ Strengthens the arms, back, butt, and neck.	■ Keep your focus upward so as not to let your head drop out of alignment. ■ Try to maintain the Swan shape throughout the exercise; don't let your head or your legs drop below your torso. ■ Don't hyperextend your low back; use your belly and your butt to tuck your pelvis under.

starting position

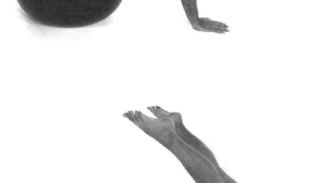

STARTING POSITION: The Plank position with hips on top of the ball, hands on the floor in front of you, fingers spread, arms strong and straight. Your legs are open and turned out in Second Position.

1 INHALE: Bend your elbows and lower your upper body toward the floor.

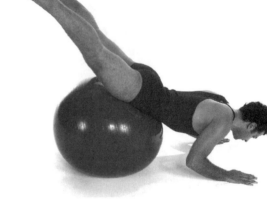

1

BENEFITS	DOS & DON'TS	IMAGINE
■ Opens the chest and reverses hunchback posture. ■ Strengthens the arms, back, butt, and neck.	■ Try to maintain the Swan shape throughout the exercise; don't let your head or your legs drop below your torso. ■ Don't hyperextend your low back; use your belly and your butt to tuck your pelvis under.	■ As you straighten your arms, imagine you are smelling a rose that sprouts from your chest.

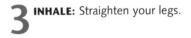

2 **EXHALE:** Bend your knees and cross your ankles, making a diamond shape with your legs. Quickly switch your ankles eight times (called *changement* in ballet).

3 **INHALE:** Straighten your legs.

4 **EXHALE:** Straighten your arms and finish with your legs open as in the start position.

repeat 4 times

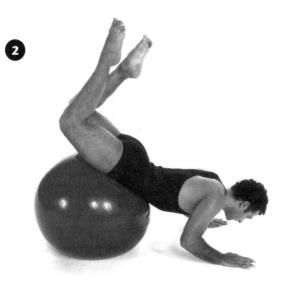

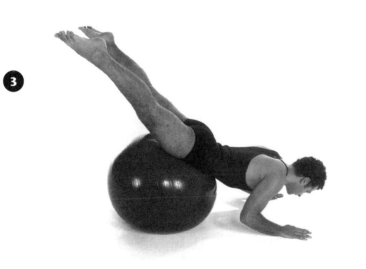

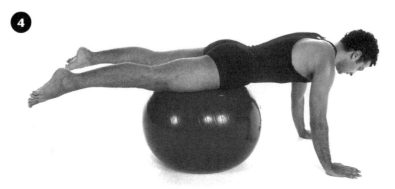

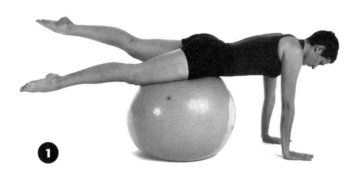

STARTING POSITION: The Plank position with hips on top of the ball, hands on the floor in front of you, fingers spread, arms strong and straight, and legs open hip distance apart, turned out from the tops of the hips.

1–2 **INHALE AND EXHALE** continuously: Keep your belly scooped up off the ball and your pubic bone pressing down on the ball as you kick your legs up and down, as when swimming, alternating legs each time.

repeat	16 times

①

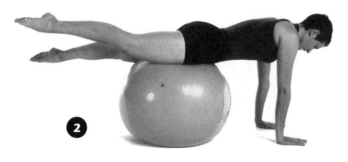

②

BENEFITS OF THE BUTT SERIES	DOS & DON'TS	IMAGINE
■ All the exercises in this series strengthen the butt and thighs.	■ Don't let the ball rock from side to side; keep the movements small and controlled. ■ Don't allow your back to arch; keep your pelvis tucked under and your butt squeezing.	■ You are anchoring the ball to the floor with your pubic bone by squeezing your butt and scooping your belly up.

charlie chaplin

1

STARTING POSITION: Start in the Plank, hips on the ball, legs straight in turn-out, feet flexed.

1 **INHALE AND EXHALE** continuously: Clap your heels together eight times. Repeat with toes pointed. Alternate every eight beats, flexing and pointing.

repeat **24 times**

heel squeezes

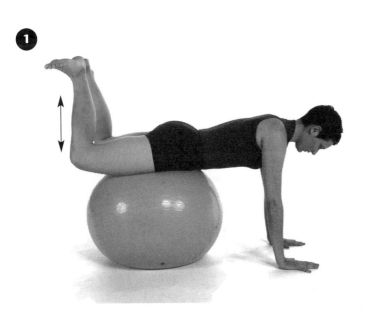

1

STARTING POSITION: Start in the Plank with hips on the ball. Open your legs wide, bend your knees, flex your feet and squeeze your heels together.

1 **INHALE AND EXHALE** continuously: On the exhale, scoop your belly up off the ball, press your pubic bone down, and pulse your thighs upward. Think of pressing up through your heels as you squeeze them together.

repeat **20 times**

butt series
scissors
intermediate

starting position

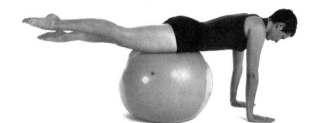

STARTING POSITION: Begin in the Plank, with legs open wide in turn-out and toes pointed.

1 **INHALE AND EXHALE** continuously: Keeping the legs straight, switch your ankles one on top of the other.

2 Vary the exercise by switching four times as you raise your legs up, and four times as you go down. (Up 2, 3, 4, and Down 2, 3, 4.)

repeat 24 times

1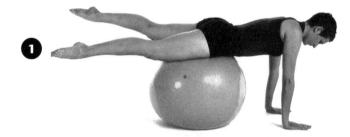

2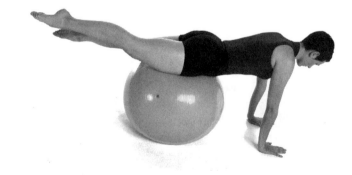

starting position

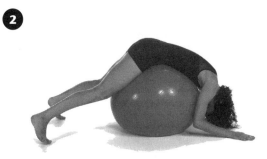

1

2

STARTING POSITION: Lie prone on the ball, hands and feet on the floor. **INHALE TO BEGIN.**

1 **EXHALE:** In one controlled yet explosive movement, extend your arms and legs up and back, and open your chest as you lift your head and upper body off the ball.

2 Come back to lying prone on the ball. **INHALE** and repeat.

repeat | 4 times

Lie on Belly Stretch: Great to do after back and butt exercises. Don't lie here longer than 30 seconds....

BENEFITS	DOS & DON'TS	IMAGINE
■ Strengthens your back, butt, and thighs. ■ Teaches balance and control.	■ Be careful! Don't be too crazy or you'll fall off the ball.	■ Your limbs are being pulled in all directions by a magnetic force.

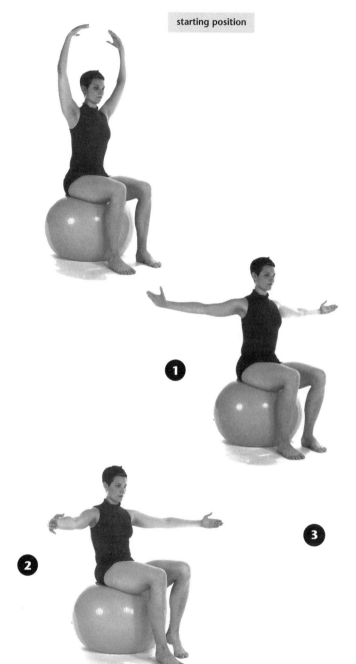

starting position

STARTING POSITION: Sit on top of the ball, feet on the floor, hip distance apart. **INHALE** as you reach your arms up to the sky.

1 Continue inhaling as you open your arms to a T.

2 **EXHALE:** As your arms come forward, scoop your belly in and slowly pull the ball forward with your tailbone, creating a C-curve in your low back.

3 Slowly walk your feet four steps forward as you roll down the ball, ending in a table top position with your hips, knees, and shoulders at the same level.

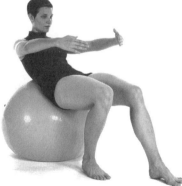

BENEFITS OF THE SUPINE SERIES	DOS & DON'TS
■ Strengthens the abdominals. ■ Teaches balance and control.	■ Go slowly so as not to roll off the ball. ■ Think of controlling the movement from the belly.

basic roll-down/roll-up

intermediate

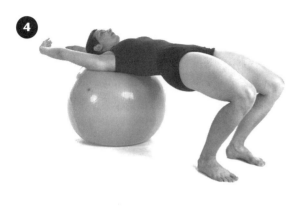

4 **INHALE:** Reach your arms up by your ears, circle them open, and then down by your sides.

5 **EXHALE:** Begin to roll back up. Start by bringing your chin to your chest and reaching your arms forward.

6 **KEEP EXHALING:** Slowly walk your feet back toward the ball four steps. Curl up until you're sitting back on top of the ball.

7 **INHALE:** Finish by sitting up tall.

repeat 6 times

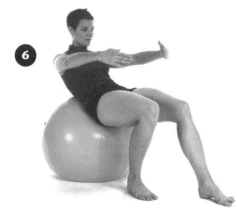

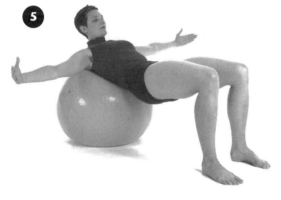

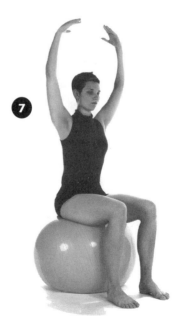

supine series

torso table top
beginning

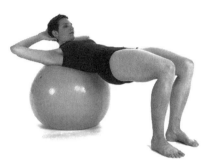

1 After the Roll-Down, stay in the table top position, keeping your hips in line with your knees and shoulders, and feet a little wider than hip distance apart, hands behind your head. Hold this position for two full inhales.

single-leg table
intermediate

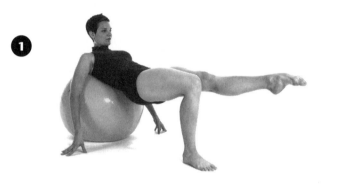

STARTING POSITION: Begin in Torso Table Top.

1 **EXHALE:** Lift one leg off the ground and straighten it forward. **INHALE** to replace it and alternate legs. You may have to put your hands on the floor to help you balance.

repeat 6 times

butt squeeze
beginning

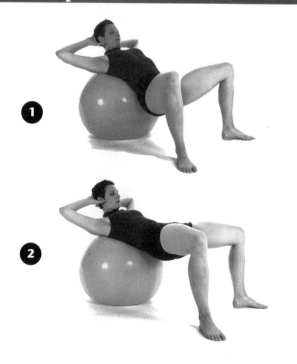

STARTING POSITION: Open your legs wide and turn your knees and feet out. Interlace your fingers and put your hands behind your head.

1 **INHALE:** Allow your butt to drop slightly.

2 **EXHALE:** Squeeze and lift your butt.

repeat 10 times

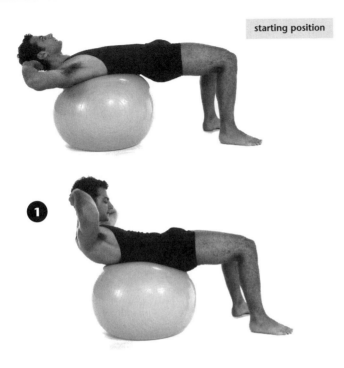

starting position

STARTING POSITION: Lie with your upper back on the ball in table top position. Your legs are wide and turned out, with hands behind your head, fingers interlaced. **INHALE TO BEGIN.**

1 EXHALE: Squeeze your butt and scoop your belly in as you curl up, Squeezing a Tangerine under your chin. Roll up so that your shoulder blades are off the ball. **INHALE** and control back down to the starting position.

repeat 8 times

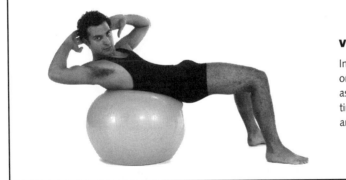

variation

Instead of curling straight up, bring one elbow toward the opposite knee as you curl up. Alternate sides 8 times or do a set of 4 on the right and 4 on the left.

BENEFITS	DOS & DON'TS	
■ Strengthens your abdominals and butt. ■ Teaches balance and control.	■ On the return, don't roll back so far that your ribcage pops up. Instead, control the movement back down to table top, keeping the ribs knitted down with your upper abs. There is no resting in this exercise, and the return is almost as hard as the curl up.	■ Don't let the hips drop as you curl up. Keep your hips as high as you can by squeezing your butt. ■ Make the exercise more challenging by starting with the ball under your lower back. When you curl up, think of pressing your low back onto the ball and deeply scooping in your belly.

starting position

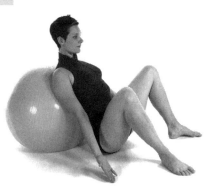

STARTING POSITION: Roll down from the table top position. Keep going so that you are in a squat, legs open and turned out, back against the ball. **INHALE TO BEGIN.**

1 EXHALE: Press into your feet, straighten your legs, and circle your arms open and then back by your ears, reaching your arms toward the floor.

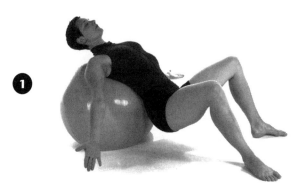

BENEFITS	DOS & DON'TS	IMAGINE
■ Stretches the belly and chest. ■ Reverses the effects of hunching over the computer (and other problems of modern life). ■ Releases the back. ■ Feels really good.	■ Don't let your feet come off the floor. You need them to stay in control. ■ Don't stay too long with your head back. You could get dizzy. ■ Don't lift your head up from the open stretch position—you could strain your neck. ■ Always return to the squat position to allow the blood to flow out of your head before trying to sit up.	■ You are floating in the Red Sea.

2 Breathe continuously in this stretch and circle your arms slowly. If you find a place in your circle that feels like it could use a good stretch, hold that place and breathe in and out. Return back to the squat and repeat.

repeat 4 times

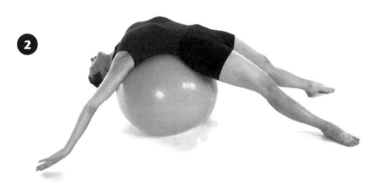

variations

Backbend
From the Lie Back Stretch position, place your hands on the floor, fingers facing toward the ball. Breathe and try to straighten your arms and legs. Return to the squat.

Backbend with single leg extension
Once in the Backbend, lift one leg off and straighten it up to the sky. Try circling it 3 times to the right, then 3 times to the left. Replace and alternate legs.

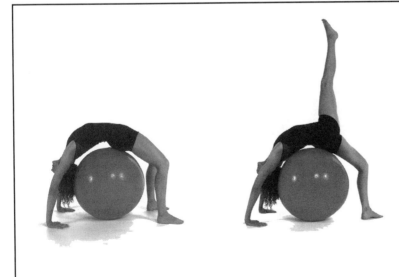

swan against the wall

starting position

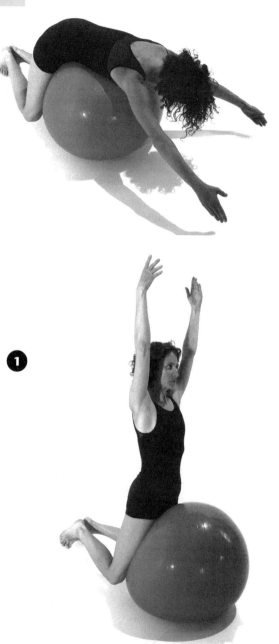

1

STARTING POSITION: Position the ball near a wall. Face away from the wall, lying prone on the ball and making sure your thighs and belly are in full contact with the ball. Your feet should be in First Position, heels squeezing together, toes apart. Press your feet firmly against the wall, especially your heels. You may have to make some adjustments with the ball before you find a stable starting point. Bring your arms by your ears.

1 **INHALE:** Press your heels into the wall as you press your thighs into the ball. Scoop your belly up off the ball and rise up into a high Swan, keeping your arms by your ears as you lift them to the sky.

BENEFITS	DOS & DON'TS	IMAGINE
■ Strengthens the hamstrings, butt, and back muscles. ■ Stretches the chest and belly. ■ Reverses hunchback posture.	■ Do initiate the movement from the core (butt and belly). ■ Don't allow the low back to arch; keep the belly scooped in and squeeze the butt to stabilize the pelvis as you open to your Swan.	■ You are a phoenix rising from the ashes.

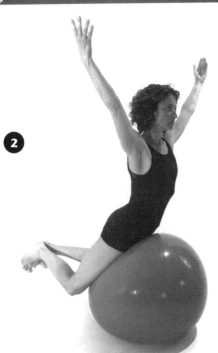

2

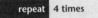

2 EXHALE: Open your arms wide.

3 INHALE: Bring your arms back up by your ears, lifting and lengthening the spine up to the heavens.

4 EXHALE: Lift your belly up as you dive back to your prone position, arms staying by the ears. Try to keep your belly so scooped that it doesn't make contact with the ball as you descend. Return to Starting Position.

repeat 4 times

3

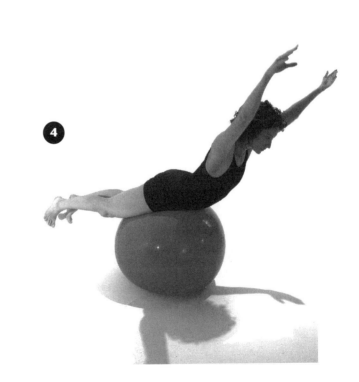

4

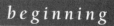
starting position

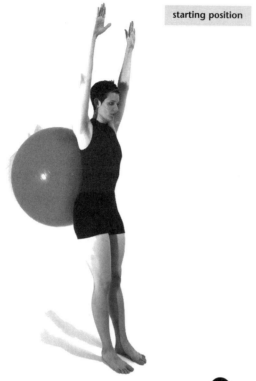

STARTING POSITION: Stand with the ball sandwiched between a wall and the small of your low back. Your knees, feet, and hips are in line with each other, and your feet are placed about 45 degrees in front of your body. **INHALE** and bring your arms up by your ears.

1 **EXHALE:** Slowly circle your arms open to a T.

1

BENEFITS	DOS & DON'TS	
■ Strengthens the legs and butt; great for skiers, snowboarders, rollerbladers, skateboarders. ■ Teaches proper knee alignment.	■ Make sure your knees do not bend too far since this can strain the joints. If you can't see your toes, you've bent too far. Walk your feet away from you if you need more space to bend your knees.	■ Don't let your knees roll open. Aim the knees over the second and third toes. ■ If you feel any discomfort in your knees, come up a little from the squat. The deeper your squat, the more strain on your knees.

2 Take your arms forward as you bend your knees as low as you can stand to, but no more than 90 degrees. Walk your feet farther away from you if you need more room. Maintain your Neutral Spine by pressing your tailbone into the ball. Press into your heels to engage the back of your legs. Hold for three full breaths. On each inhale, start a new arm circle by bringing your arms up by your ears, completing the circle on the exhale. (These arm circles are a great way to distract yourself from the pain in your legs.) Come back up to straight legs.

repeat 3 times

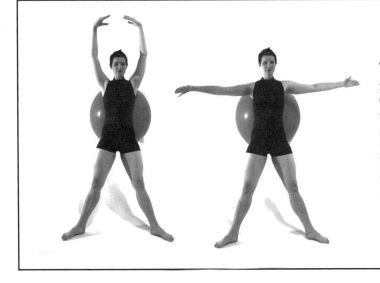

variation 2nd Position

Second Position: Start with your legs open wide and turned out (knees facing away from each other). Again, to maintain proper knee alignment, make sure the knees are aimed over the second and third toes. A common mistake in this position is allowing the knees to roll in.
Reverse the direction of the arm circle.

part three:

cool down

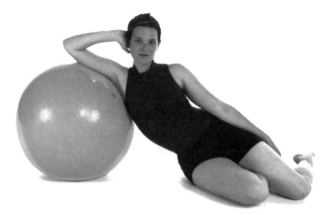

STARTING POSITION: Sit on the side of your hip with your knees bent, legs folded on top of each other, and your top leg in back. Put one hand on the side of your head and lean the side of your ribs and your armpit against the ball. Let your other arm rest in front of you or on your legs. Breathe continuously for approximately 30 seconds, allowing your ribcage to drop down toward the floor. If you don't feel a side stretch, then move the ball a little away from you.

BENEFITS	DOS & DON'TS	IMAGINE
■ Stretches the side body, specifically the oblique abdominals and the quadratus lumborum.	■ Do enjoy the stretch. ■ Make sure to take deep breaths to fully get the benefits of this stretch.	■ You are a bathing beauty of a bygone era.

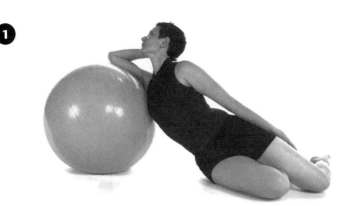

1 Slowly roll your upper body back, allowing your back to arch. Breathe in this stretch.

2 Slowly roll the ball forward, allowing the low back to round, keeping your belly scooped in. Breathe in this stretch.

3 To complete the full twist, scoop your belly in and reach your top knee forward. Reach your back arm onto the ball behind you to secure the upper body. Breathe.

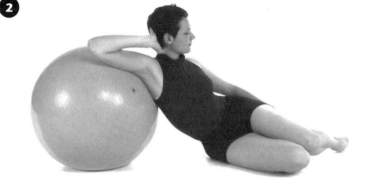

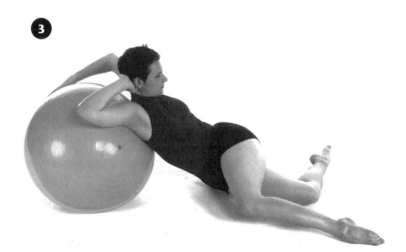

starting position

STARTING POSITION: Kneel with the ball in front of you, hands on top of the ball, arms straight. Think of gently squeezing your butt to push your hips forward, tucking your pelvis under. **INHALE TO BE-GIN.**

1 EXHALE: Begin "the wave" by dropping your head forward as if you are diving under water.

2 Peel down your spine one vertebra at a time, and allow the ball to slowly roll forward with your hands.

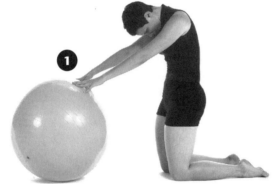

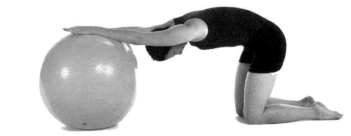

BENEFITS	DOS & DON'TS	IMAGINE
■ Stretches and articulates the spine. ■ Strengthens the butt, hamstrings, and belly.	■ Keep your butt in line with your knees as you roll down and back up your spine; this takes work in the butt, hamstrings, and belly.	■ You are a cat waking up after a nap in the afternoon sun.

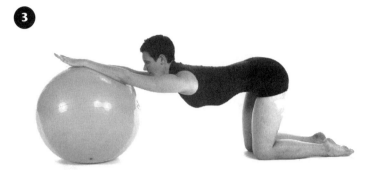

3 **INHALE:** "Come up for air" as you arch your back, stick your butt out a little to really get a cat stretch in your spine. Let your eyes look upward toward the sky, and allow your armpits to gently drop down toward the floor, stretching your shoulders.

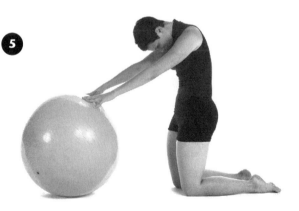

4–6 **EXHALE:** Retrograde the movement to return to the starting position. Begin by tucking your tail under, scooping your belly in and stacking your spine one vertebra at a time until you return to starting position.

repeat 3 times

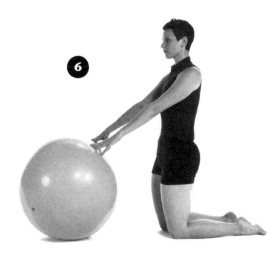

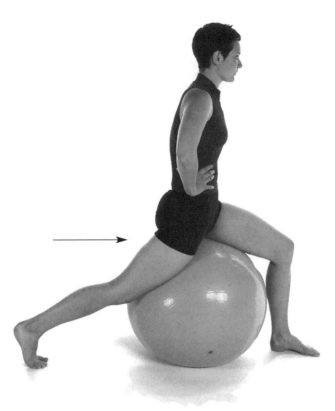

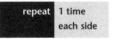

STARTING POSITION: Get into a lunge position with the ball between your legs, so that you are gently sitting on it. Both legs should be bent; the forward leg has a flat foot so you can stabilize and bear weight. Press into the ball of the back foot, allowing the heel to lift off the floor. **INHALE TO BEGIN.**

1 **EXHALE:** Scoop your belly in and squeeze your butt as the back thigh squeezes the ball. Tuck your pelvis under and feel the stretch in the front of your hip. Hold the stretch for 30 seconds and switch sides.

repeat	1 time each side

BENEFITS	DOS & DON'TS
■ Stretches your psoas and hip flexors.	■ Do take the arch out of your back. ■ Keep your belly pulled in.

starting position

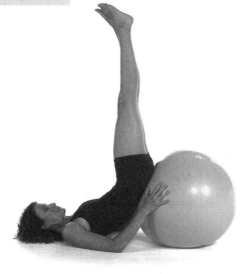

STARTING POSITION: Lie on your back, legs up in the air, holding the ball right in front of your butt. Levitate your hips up to the sky and, using your glutes and abdominals, pull the ball underneath your hips.

1 Drop one leg forward onto the ball and let the other knee drop toward your chest. Breathing deeply, tuck your pelvis under and use your hamstrings and glutes to squeeze the ball with your heel, which will increase the stretch in the front of your hip. Hold for 30 seconds.

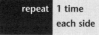

repeat | 1 time each side

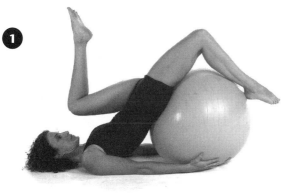

BENEFITS	DOS & DON'TS
■ Stretches psoas and hip flexors. ■ Strengthens glutes and hamstrings.	■ Don't roll onto your neck. Instead, balance on your shoulder blades.

index

books by ulysses press

ASHTANGA YOGA FOR WOMEN:
INVIGORATING MIND, BODY, AND SPIRIT WITH POWER YOGA
Sally Griffyn, $17.95
Presents the exciting and empowering practice of power yoga in a balanced fashion that addresses the specific needs of female practitioners.

ELLLIE HERMAN'S PILATES MATWORK PROPS WORKBOOK:
STEP-BY-STEP GUIDE WITH OVER 200 PHOTOS
Ellie Herman, $12.95
This book explains how props can enhance Pilates in its own way: the magic circles tone arms, the small ball held between the legs shapes thighs, the foam roller stretches the chest and shoulders, and the large exercise ball builds core stability.

THE JOSEPH H. PILATES METHOD AT HOME: A BALANCE, SHAPE, STRENGTH & FITNESS PROGRAM
Eleanor McKenzie, $16.95
This handbook describes and details Pilates, a mental and physical program that combines elements of yoga and classical dance.

PILATES PERSONAL TRAINER BACK STRENGTHENING WORKOUT:
ILLUSTRATED STEP-BY-STEP MATWORK ROUTINE
Michael King and Yolande Green, $9.95
The easy starter program in this workbook teaches Pilates exercises that are appropriate for strengthening the back in a safe and healthy manner.

PILATES PERSONAL TRAINER GETTING STARTED WITH STRETCHING:
ILLUSTRATED STEP-BY-STEP MATWORK ROUTINE
Michael King and Yolande Green, $9.95
Ideal for beginners or older people, the specially designed Pilates exercises in this book offer a gentle workout of light strength movements and key stretches.

PILATES PERSONAL TRAINER POWERHOUSE ABS WORKOUT:
ILLUSTRATED STEP-BY-STEP MATWORK ROUTINE
Michael King and Yolande Green, $9.95
Designed for those who want to flatten and shape their abs, this book explains each Pilates exercise in an easy-to-follow manner. The key element is the series of two-page, step-by-step photo sequences that illustrate and demonstrate each exercise.

PILATES PERSONAL TRAINER THIGHS & BUTT WORKOUT:
ILLUSTRATED STEP-BY-STEP MATWORK ROUTINE
Michael King and Yolande Green, $9.95
Instead of paying $100-plus per hour for private Pilates sessions, those looking to get the same kind of targeted workout to shape and slim their thighs and buttocks can find it in this book.

PILATES WORKBOOK:
ILLUSTRATED STEP-BY-STEP GUIDE TO MATWORK TECHNIQUES
Michael King, $12.95
Illustrates the core matwork movements exactly as Joseph Pilates intended them to be performed; readers learn each movement by following the photographic sequences and explanatory captions.

PILATES WORKBOOK FOR PREGNANCY:
ILLUSTRATED STEP-BY-STEP MATWORK TECHNIQUES
Michael King and Yolande Green, $12.95
Presented in an easy-to-use style with step-by-step photo sequences of Pilates matwork techniques—adapted here for pregnancy and post-pregnancy.

SENSES WIDE OPEN: THE ART & PRACTICE OF LIVING IN YOUR BODY
Johanna Putnoi, $14.95
Through simple, accessible exercises, this book shows how to be at ease with yourself and experience genuine pleasure in your physical connection to others and the world.

YOGA IN FOCUS: POSTURES, SEQUENCES, AND MEDITATIONS
Jessie Chapman   photographs by Dhyan, $14.95
A beautiful celebration of yoga that's both useful for learning the techniques and inspiring in its artistic approach to presenting the body in yoga positions.

YOGA FOR PARTNERS: OVER 75 POSTURES TO DO TOGETHER
Jessie Chapman   photographs by Dhyan, $14.95
An excellent tool for learning two-person yoga, Yoga for Partners features inspiring photos of the paired asanas. It teaches each partner how to synchronize their movements and breathing, bringing new lightness and enjoyment to any yoga practice.

YOGA THERAPIES: 45 SEQUENCES TO RELIEVE STRESS, DEPRESSION,
REPETITIVE STRAIN, SPORTS INJURIES AND MORE
Jessie Chapman   photographs by Dhyan, $14.95
Featuring an inspiring artistic presentation, this book is filled with beautifully photographed sequences that relieve stress, release anger, relax back muscles and reverse repetitive strain injuries.

To order these books call 800-377-2542 or 510-601-8301, fax 510-601-8307, e-mail ulysses@ ulyssespress.com, or write to Ulysses Press, P.O. Box 3440, Berkeley, CA 94703. All retail orders are shipped free of charge. California residents must include sales tax. Allow two to three weeks for delivery.

about the models

Dano Gregori received his formal Pilates training at Ellie Herman Studios in San Francisco. He is a rehabilitation specialist using the work of Janda and myofascial release techniques. His private and group classes provide a challenging training environment with focus on stability and alignment. Dano has a background in psychology, Chi Nei Tsang (Taoist Internal Organ Massage), and naturopathy. For information about his Palm Springs Studio see www.danogregori.com.

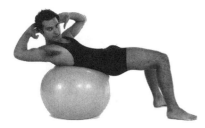

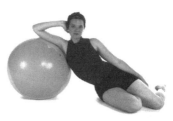

Alisa Michelle, originally from Toronto, Canada, began her Pilates training at The School of Toronto Dance Theater and The Studio. Upon moving to San Francisco, she began her studies at the Ellie Herman Studios, where she completed the Pilates Intensive Training Program. Alisa teaches Pilates at Ellie Herman Studios, Sanchez St. Studios, and Gold's Gym. She is also currently directing as well as dancing for Company Mecanique Dance Theater.

about the photographer

Andy Mogg specializes in dance photography in the San Francisco Bay Area. Portraiture, headshots, videography, and wedding services are also provided by his company, Dancing Images. For more information visit www.dancingimages.com.